THE ART AND SCIENCE OF THYROID SUPPLEMENTATION FOR THE TREATMENT OF BIPOLAR DEPRESSION

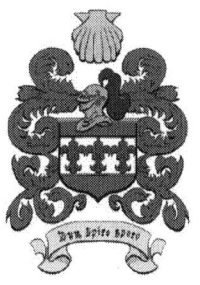

TAMMAS KELLY, MD

Director: The Depression & Bipolar Clinic of Colorado

Associate Clinical Professor
The George Washington University School of Medicine and Health Sciences Department of Psychiatry and Behavioral Sciences
Washington DC

© 2017 Tammas Kelly, MD
All rights reserved.

ISBN: 1979168415
ISBN 13: 9781979168410
Library of Congress Control Number: **XXXXX (If applicable)**
LCCN Imprint Name: **City and State (If applicable)**

Manic depression is a frustrating

mess

–Jimi Hendrix

Acknowledgments I would like to thank first and foremost the chair at University of Miami Department of Psychiatry & Behavioral Sciences Charlie Nemeroff. Charlie started me on this journey with his admonition to keep going up on the thyroid dose. Without him I would have never discovered the benefits of high dose thyroid for my patients. I have built much on the work of professors Michael Bauer and Peter Whybrow done at UCLA and later at Technische Universität Dresden. These are two giant's shoulders that I surely stand upon. I would also thank Professors Steven Dubovsky, Hagop Akiskal and Nassir Ghaemi who have all taken me under their wing, encouraged and mentored my research. Jim Phelps MD of PsychEducation.org fame, has also mentored me and encouraged me. Jim has no peer in the world for knowledge of bipolar spectrum disorders. He has been the key to my understanding of the bipolar disorders. Without him we still be in the stone age in our understanding of the bipolar spectrum disorders. My greatest mentor has been Prof. Daniel Lieberman who has co-authored many of my papers. He has taught me much about the science of psychiatry despite his strange fetish for piñatas. George Washington University Department of Psychiatry and Behavioral Sciences and the chair James Griffith deserve special acknowledgment for providing me with the resources to do my research. Lastly, I would thank Lanny Douglas APRN and Rabbi Dr. Larry Denmark along with Jim Phelps and Daniel Lieberman who have tirelessly reviewed, edited and made suggestions for the book and other publications. Chris Akens MD and Gary Sachs MD also pitched in with some helpful suggestions.

Table of Contents

PART I
Intro and Quick Guide to the Use of High Dose Thyroid

CHAPTER ONE
Introduction to the Use Thyroid Hormones to Treat Bipolar Disorders 1

CHAPTER TWO
A Quick Guide to the Practical Use of High-Dose Thyroid.........8

CHAPTER THREE
Important Definitions...32

PART II
The Evidence Base of the Efficacy and Safety of High Dose Thyroid

Chapter Four
Why HDT Isn't Hyperthyroidism..36

Chapter Five
Evidence That HDT Works and Works Well..............................42

Chapter Six
The Myth That HDT Causes Osteoporosis................................52

Chapter Seven
The Myth That High-Dose Thyroid Is a Cardiac Risk Factor.....65

Chapter Eight
The Risks of Other Psychiatric Medications and the Undertreatment of Bipolar Disorders..75

Chapter Nine
Is HDT A Risk Factor for Mania?............................87

Chapter Ten
The Use of HDT During Pregnancy and Breastfeeding............90

Chapter Eleven
T3 vs. T4..95

Chapter Twelve
Unique Aspects of HDT..102

Chapter Thirteen
The Theory of How Thyroid Hormone Works in Treatment of Bipolar Disorders....................................107

Part III
The Politics of High Dose Thyroid

Chapter Fourteen
Post Hoc Ergo Propter Hoc: Where the Field of Endocrinology Went Wrong..116

Chapter Fifteen
Psychiatrists' Role as Specialists...........................126

Chapter Sixteen
Summation..130

Appendix
    Abbreviations..135

    Patient Information Handout..............................136

    Model Letter to Physicians Involved in the Treatment of Your Patient..140

References..144

Chapter 1: Introduction to the Use Thyroid Hormones to Treat Bipolar Disorders

If the use of high doses of thyroid makes you nervous, publish it and let the world decide.

—Advice to the author from Mark Frye, MD, Chair, Psychiatry and Psychology

Mayo Clinic

One half of what you were taught as medical students will in 10 years have been shown to be wrong, and the trouble is, your teachers don't know which half.

—C. Sidney Burwell (1893–1967) *British Medical Journal* 2, 113, 1956

A universal experience in medical school is the feeling of disbelief when it is disclosed that within ten years, half of what we are learning will be wrong. This is as true now as it was in 1956. This book presents clear and convincing evidence of one important "fact" that is just starting to gain acceptance. That is that high dose thyroid (HDT) does not cause the medical sequela associated with hyperthyroidism. That HDT does not cause the same sequela as hyperthyroidism is met with almost universal disbelief—to the point that many will refuse to consider the evidence that will be presented in this book. Yet to reject this conclusion without examining the literature is an anathema to the practice of evidence-based medicine and a failure to consider C. Sidney Burwell's maxim that our knowledge base in medicine is ever changing.

High dose thyroid (HDT) works and works well for controlling bipolar depression and is recommended in multiple bipolar treatment guidelines. Often, it is key to reaching euthymia.

Despite this, HDT is largely overlooked as a treatment primarily because of the mistaken idea that it causes hyperthyroidism. By the end of the book, you should be able to understand why asking what the risks are of high dose thyroid (HDT) use may not be as important as asking what the risks are of *not* using HDT. This book is a primer on the safe, evidenced-based use of HDT to treat bipolar disorders; it will give the reader everything needed to start prescribing HDT with confidence. This book discusses the art and science of using HDT to treat the bipolar disorders.

There is very little research on how to treat bipolar I depression and almost a total absence of research on how to treat bipolar II/NOS depressions. With such a dearth of research, we need to use every treatment option available. We need to pay special attention to "orphan" medications—i.e. medications that do not have the financial backing of a drug company.

I became interested in HDT 20 years ago, out of sheer desperation born of a having practice with a large number of patients suffering from bipolar depression. In other words, I had many patients who were not doing well. I presented a particularly refractory case to Dr. Charlie Nemeroff, then chair of the Emory Department of Psychiatry. He questioned why I never went beyond 50 mcg of T3. I mumbled something barely articulate that 50 mcg was as high as I was taught to go but no higher.

He said in a loud, supportive voice, "No. Keep going up. Keep going up!"

I proceeded to slowly raise the dose of T3. It didn't help, not at all—at least for the patient that I had presented. However, it did work for most of my other bipolar patients.

With the regular use of HDT, I came under heavy criticism from endocrinologists and other physicians. My reaction was to review the literature in order to develop an accurate risk-benefit analysis for HDT. This book is the product of that search. The scientific support for the statements made in this chapter will be developed later in the book. My bias was that HDT would carry a significant risk. Like most doctors, I assumed that HDT caused hyperthyroidism, placing the patient at risk for osteoporosis and a myriad of cardiovascular risks. The primary questions were: How did the risks of HDT compare with the risks of other medications, and how did the risks of HDT compare with failing to fully stabilize a patient's bipolar disorder? Much to my astonishment, I found that HDT is not the same as hyperthyroidism, and no quality research showed a significant risk from HDT. The few studies that do indicate that HDT may carry some medical risks are so badly flawed that they could not be counted as definitive evidence. These studies, when carefully evaluated, indicated that HDT is safe rather than the opposite. There is no question that hyperthyroidism and even subclinical hyperthyroidism carry significant morbidity and mortality. However, when one examines just the literature regarding the use of HDT, as defined here as > 50 mcg of T3 or > 200 mcg of T4, there is overwhelming support that it does not equate with hyperthyroidism and that it is safe. The cause of the physical damage from hyperthyroidism is not known, but it is suspected that it is more likely related to autoimmune mechanisms than to the direct effects of high circulating levels of thyroid hormone.

Another surprising fact is that most of the research showing that HDT is safe comes directly from the field of endocrinology. Endocrinologists routinely recommended HDT to prevent the recurrence of thyroid cancer. The risk of recurrence of thyroid cancer—at least stages II, III, and IV thyroid cancer—carries less mortality than the bipolar disorders do. Further, the bipolar disorders carry much more morbidity than any stage of thyroid cancer does. I was startled to find that the clear and universally accepted definition of hyperthyroidism could not be applied to HDT. HDT doesn't even fit the definition of thyrotoxicosis. To be sure, too much thyroid hormone can cause thyrotoxicosis even in patients with a bipolar disorder, but in general, when using HDT to treat a bipolar disorder, if toxic symptoms develop, the dose of thyroid is decreased.

Why Doesn't HDT Fit the Definition of Hyperthyroidism?

Hyperthyroidism is defined as the overproduction of endogenous thyroid hormone with accompanying signs and symptoms of thyrotoxicosis. Thyrotoxicosis is defined as the presence of signs and symptoms of high circulating levels of thyroid hormone. Both definitions require confirmation by laboratory studies of the high level of thyroid hormone. Subclinical hyperthyroidism is a type of hyperthyroidism. Subclinical hyperthyroidism is defined as low TSH with normal T3 and T4 levels. Some definitions allow for some thyrotoxic symptoms; others do not. HDT fails to fit the definition of hyperthyroidism on two points. First, the high circulating levels of thyroid hormone are exogenous; and second, the dosing of high-dose thyroid is kept at a level low enough not to cause thyrotoxic symptoms. By these definitions, references citing HDT as causing hyperthyroidism are erroneous. HDT is often identified as iatrogenic hyperthyroidism, which, by definition, is an oxymoron stemming from a post hoc, ergo propter hoc error. That is, correlation is mistaken for causation. We've been operating under the mistaken idea that because high circulating levels of thyroid hormones cause thyrotoxic symptoms and are correlated with the medical sequela of hyperthyroidism, the high circulating levels of hormone must be the direct cause of the medical sequela of hyperthyroidism. Some endocrinologists have accused me of splitting hairs, yet the large body of evidence from HDT treatment research demonstrates an absence of morbidity and mortality. A review of this literature strongly supports the conclusion that high circulating levels of thyroid hormone do not directly cause the medical sequela of hyperthyroidism.

Hyperthyroidism is an autoimmune disorder. It appears most likely that the autoimmune cascade is the factor causing the medical sequela. A number of the medical sequela of hyperthyroidism have already been proven to be caused by an autoimmune process, for example, exophthalmos and Graves' pretibial myxedema (Topliss and Eastman, 2004; Wall and Lahooti, 2010). There is mounting evidence that many of the other of the sequelae of hyperthyroidism are caused by an autoimmune processes (Biondi and Kahaly, 2010). These autoimmune problems persist even after ablation of the thyroid gland (Laurberg et al., 2008; Ponto et al., 2010). It is the ongoing presence of these autoimmune factors that excludes for consideration any research into the safety of HDT that involves patients who are or have been hyperthyroid (including subclinical hypothyroidism). Endocrinologists have failed to recognize this and therefore have built up a mythos surrounding HDT.

This book explores and dispels the myths of HDT. These myths include:

1. HDT equates with hyperthyroidism.
2. HDT causes osteoporosis.
3. HDT carries significant cardiovascular risks.
4. High circulating levels of thyroid hormone are the cause of the medical sequela of hyperthyroidism.

I will show evidence that HDT is effective and as safe as or safer than many of the other medicines commonly used to treat bipolar disorders.

In addition, I will discuss the possibility that HDT has some unique properties that may be particularly helpful to patients suffering from a bipolar disorder. That is, HDT can significantly decrease the cognitive problems associated with the bipolar disorders, and HDT could significantly decrease the considerable medical morbidity and mortality associated with the bipolar disorders, which cause our patients' premature deaths more frequently than suicide does.

Aside from psychotherapy, HDT is the oldest psychiatric treatment in continuous use that is still in use today. The use of thyroid hormones to treat affective disorders dates back to at least 1899 where the Emil Kraepelin lectured about the use of desiccated sheep thyroids (Kraepelin, 1899).

Although it predated the introduction of electroconvulsive therapy (ECT) by nearly a decade, the use of HDT to treat the bipolar disorders remains largely ignored despite a large number of studies showing that it is efficacious (Bauer et al., 2003; Bauer et al., 2002; Bauer et al., 2015; Bauer et al., 2005; Bauer and Whybrow, 2001; Bauer and Whybrow, 1990; Kelly and Lieberman, 2009). Perhaps the highest-quality data showing efficacy of HDT comes from a randomized, double-blind, placebo-controlled study.

Further, HDT has been repeatedly shown to normalize brain function in neuroimaging studies (Bauer et al., 2015; Bauer et al., 2005). HDT is ignored despite the fact that its use has been recommended by published treatment guidelines since 2000, including the Expert Consensus Guideline Series Medication Treatment of Bipolar Disorder, the American Psychiatric

Association bipolar treatment guidelines, the most up-to-date Canadian bipolar treatment guidelines (2013), and the Texas Algorithm Project bipolar guidelines (Crismon et al., 2007; Hirschfeld, 2010; Sachs et al., 2000; Yatham et al., 2013).

HDT is not a panacea. It doesn't work for all, nor does it work as a monotherapy.

The learning curve to use HDT is comparable to learning how to use lithium (Li). With so few psychiatrists using HDT, there is a risk that the clinical wisdom and pragmatic know-how necessary to use HDT could be lost. By clinical wisdom, I mean **the collective body of experience not found in scientific literature that develops with extensive use of a medication and/or gets passed down from generation to generation of psychiatrists**.

The purpose of this book is to pass on the clinical wisdom of HDT as well as to review the research showing that HDT is effective and safe. The clinical wisdom includes which patients are likely to respond to HDT, what side effects to expect, how to deal with those side effects, the best starting dose, how to increase the dose, at what dose should you start to see improvement, at what dose can you conclude that HDT is not going to work, how to combine HDT with other treatments, what to expect from HDT in the long run, and how to get the most out of HDT.

This book will be divided into three sections, the "quick-start guide," the evidence base section, and a discussion section. The quick-start guide contains practical advice based both on the science and on thirty years of experience using thyroid to treat affective disorders. (The first 10 years were with doses of T3 50 mcg or less.) It discusses the nitty-gritty of using HDT and is designed to find quick answers and practical solutions. The science section provides the needed evidence to practice safe, evidence-based medicine. It will address the following: the evidence showing the efficacy of HDT, the safety of HDT, that HDT is not equivalent to hyperthyroidism, the safety of HDT compared with other medications, which thyroid hormone is best (T3 or T4), and the safety of HDT during pregnancy and breastfeeding. The discussion section will give helpful information for dealing with those who oppose the use of HDT and discuss the proposed hypothesis of how HDT works.

This primer will not be the final word on the use of HDT. Much research has yet to be done.

Chapter 2: A Quick Guide to the Practical Use of High-Dose Thyroid

In theory there is no difference between theory and practice. In practice there is.

—Yogi Berra

This chapter is designed as a quick-reference guide. The scientific support will come in the following chapters. At first glance, these instructions may seem a bit intimidating. High-dose thyroid (HDT) has a learning curve larger than Lithium. Selective serotonin reuptake inhibitors. do but less than lithium does. The instructions follow common-sense medical principles or are extensions of existing medical knowledge.

Who Should Get a Trial of High-Dose Thyroid?

1. Any affectively ill patient who has been refractory to early treatments.
2. Any patient experiencing rapid-cycling
3. Any affectively ill patient who has failed to reach full and complete remission. Residual affective disorders have a large impact on patients, their families, and society at large. Residual symptoms can still be devastating, and incomplete remission puts the patient at risk for severe relapses.
4. All bipolar patients? There are some theoretical reasons to believe that for patients who see benefits from HDT, HDT may lessen the medical mortality and morbidity associated with the bipolar disorders. See chapters 4, 5, 6, 8, and 13.

Starting HDT

HDT will not work alone. It needs to be added to other medications used to stabilize the bipolar disorders. It can be combined safely with any presently known psychiatric medication. HDT can be used successfully with all mood stabilizers, stimulants, N-acetyl cysteine, dextromethorphan/quinidine, typical antipsychotics, atypical antipsychotics (including Clozaril), pramipexole, benzodiazepines, modafinil, armodafinil, lithium, donepezil, beta blockers, and yes, even antidepressants (including MAOIs, Saint John's wort, and SAME). HDT does not appear to clash with any over-the-counter medications.

Clinically, the recommendation is to use T3 (see the chapter on T3 vs. T4). T4 or Armour Thyroid and similar products can be successfully used, but they take longer to reach an optimum dose, and the risk for side effects (discussed below) is higher, due to the longer half-life. Any form of thyroid preparation will work, but there are valid reasons to choose T3. If T4 is to be used, substitute 100 mcg of T4 = 25 mcg of T3.

1. The goal is to find the dose that achieves maximum symptom relief with minimal side effects.
2. *For bipolar I patients only*: the initial goal is to bring T3 into the high normal range and TSH into the low normal range. This is often enough. This is the only time that thyroid levels can be useful. For bipolar II/NOS, this approach doesn't work. If a patient with bipolar I does not respond to this approach, then keep increasing the dose as discussed below.
3. Start with 25 mcg of T3 and increase the dose 25 mcg each week until initial benefit is seen.
4. When increasing the dose, see the patient every two weeks to monitor for pulse and side effects.
5. There will be times that it is advisable to see patients more often or increase the dose only by 12.5 mcg per week.
6. If patients are unwilling or unable to return in two weeks, then increase the dose by 25 mcg and increase it another 25 mcg the week before they come in.
7. If the dose of T3 reaches 125 mcg without benefit, it is advisable to increase the dose 12.5 mcg per week and/or see the patient weekly.
8. Instruct the patient that if he or she experiences a significant side effect to decrease the dose by 25 mcg and wait until the next appointment to discuss what to do. To prevent premature discontinuation, emphasize to the patient that he or she should not decrease the dose further without discussing it with you.

9. Instruct the patient to stop increasing T3 when he or she experiences improvement. The dose likely will need to be adjusted upward, but by 12.5 mcg each week, to facilitate finding the optimum dose.

What medications can HDT be safely used with? The short answer is that it can be combined with any known psychiatric treatment.

Preparing the Patient to Take HDT

1. **Safety**: The single biggest issue holding back the use of HDT has been the greatly overblown concern about its safety. To sum up the whole issue: HDT is as safe as or safer than many of our psychiatric medications (see chapter 8). Explain this to the patient ahead of time because inevitably, someone will become upset about the HDT.
2. **Treatment guidelines**: Inform the patient that HDT is recommended in many bipolar treatment guidelines.
3. **Other doctors**: It is important to inform the patient at the outset that his or her other doctors may have less knowledge about HDT. Explain to the patient that it isn't because they are bad doctors but because the amount of medical information has become so vast that it is difficult for family physicians and specialists in different fields to be fully knowledgeable of every area of medicine. Explain that the other doctors disagree only because they are not familiar with the scientific research available and are unaware that HDT is recommended in bipolar treatment guidelines.
    a. Send other doctors involved in the patient's care a copy of the thyroid letter found in the appendix, and give a copy to the patient.
    b. Instruct patients to carry a copy of the letter next to their list of medications so that it is available to show future doctors. This is especially important if a patient ends up in the emergency room.

     c. Instruct patients that if another doctor wants to decrease their thyroid dose, both the other physician and the patient need to talk to you first.
4. **Time of improvement**: It is critically important to frame patient expectations of how long it may take to start to see improvement. Explain that most patients will start to respond at somewhere between 50 mcg and 125 mcg of T3. Occasionally some patients will respond to lower doses, and some need a dose well beyond 125 mcg. Depending on how aggressive you are in increasing the dose of T3, patients will often feel frustrated if, five to six weeks out, they have experienced no improvement. It is best to tell patients that they will experience frustration at the outset. As long as the patient is not experiencing side effects, there is no reason *not* to keep increasing the dose until you see improvement or side effects. Keep in mind that enzyme-inducing agents such as carbamazepine or oxcarbazepine will require higher doses of thyroid hormone because of first pass effects in the liver.
5. **Patient frustration**: When patients do get frustrated and want to quit, remind them that because of the time it takes for some patients to reach a therapeutic dose, it was predictable that they would become frustrated and that this is normal. Acknowledge to the patent that the situation is frustrating but (this is critically important) emphasize that it is not frustrating for you, the doctor. Using the metaphor of swimming three quarters of the way across a river, getting tired, and deciding to swim back can be helpful. Remind patients that if they quit now, they may find themselves having to go through this all over again in the future, starting from scratch, so it is best to complete the HDT trial.
6. **Stopping HDT**: Discuss what will happen if the patient needs to stop the thyroid hormone for any reason.
     a. Doses of 50 mcg or less can be stopped abruptly, generally without a problem. At higher doses, it is best to taper down the thyroid hormone slowly, lowering the dose by 12.5 to 25 mcg every one to two weeks. A slow taper allows the

patient's thyroid gland to slowly take over production. Most importantly, when the hormone is tapered slowly, emerging bipolar symptoms are usually easier to deal with.
  b. If the thyroid hormone has been helpful, warn the patient that he or she is likely to relapse and that it might not happen right away. Often the relapse will happen within a couple days of the first one or two dosage decreases. Interestingly, even T4 decreases can bring on relapses within a day or two after reduction. At other times, relapse may be delayed by month or longer.
  c. Warn patients that they may feel better—in fact, they may feel great—and that this could be the start of hypomania or mania.
  d. If a patient is stopping T3 because he or she has seen no improvement or is feeling worse, see the section below, When and How to Decide That Thyroid Hormone Is Not Going to Work.
7. **Review current medical problems**: If patients have significant heart problems, consider how an increase in heart rate may affect that condition. Likely, the heart rate will go up with HDT. Keep in mind that just as with all medications, the older a patient is, the higher the risk for side effects or adverse reactions. Age alone cannot guide you. HDT in the elderly can be less risky than the alternative medications. (See chapter 8, risks.)
8. **Major side effects to be discussed** (see table 1): It is important to emphasize that side effects are generally minimal and usually easily handled by decreasing the dose of thyroid.
  a. **Sudden increase in anxiety.** It is very important to tell the patient first that HDT can be very helpful in decreasing anxiety, but like a number of other medications, too much can *cause* anxiety—for example, akathisia from neuroleptics. If you start by telling a patient that it might cause anxiety, you will spend the next

ten minutes explaining why he or she should try it despite the risk of anxiety.
  b. **Increased heart rate.** Explain to the patient that in general, it is best to keep the resting heart rate below 100. Explain that a resting heart rate is when the patient is relaxed and hasn't had any vigorous physical activity for at least 30 minutes.
  c. **Feeling too warm or hot**. Too much thyroid can increase the metabolism to the point where patients are overheating. This sometimes comes in the form of hot flashes. Some patients are hot all the time. If the patient is uncomfortable, he or she is getting too much thyroid, and it is time to decrease the dose. There are some caveats, such as if the patient is only experiencing hot flashes at night. See how to handle side effects below.
9. Rarely, perhaps one patient in 200 will experience **excruciating bone and joint pains** at 25 or 50 mcg of T3. This is generally in the hands and feet. Instruct the patient that if this happens, he or she should stop thyroid altogether. Patients won't have to guess if this is happening. This is not to be mistaken for the milder, dose-dependent, bone and joint pains that can occur at the higher doses. See side effect section below.
10. **Consider caffeine use**: It is absolutely amazing how much caffeine some patients use. Ask how many cups patients are drinking and how big the cups are. In the last 30 years a cup of coffee has gone from six ounces to 16 (or more). Caffeine potentiates the heart rate of patients taking HDT. It may increase the risk of atrial fibrillation. For heart rates above 100, see side effect discussion below. The thing to tell the patient is that HDT will eventually help with energy and motivation more than caffeine does. Ask the patient to consider cutting back on caffeine. If the heart rate is above ninety, inform the patient that the thyroid dose cannot be increased unless he or she cuts back on caffeine or stops using it.

Follow-up Appointments

Schedule follow-up visits after every dose increase or, if the patient is stable, every three to four months. Discuss the following:

1. **Ask about side effects.** Distinguish between minor side effects and bothersome side effects. See how to handle side effects below.
2. **Monitor heart rate.** Use a pulse oximeter that has a wave form. The wave form is very helpful for detecting an irregularly irregular heartbeat, the hallmark of atrial fibrillation. Pulse oximeter can be found on the Internet for $50-60 Alternatively, a one-lead EKG can be used. One-lead EKGs are relatively inexpensive, $80, and are reimbursable by insurance. Search for AliveCor. If you think you can detect atrial fibrillation by palpation of the pulse, more power to you. But it takes longer and is not as accurate. If the heart rate is between 90 and 100, inform the patient that the thyroid dose cannot be increased unless he or she cuts back on caffeine. For heart rate > 100, see side effect discussion below.

When and How to Decide That Thyroid Hormone Is Not Going to Work

Thyroid hormone should be increased until the patient either has symptom relief or side effects. If no benefits are seen in the face of clearly identified side effects, then the thyroid hormone should be slowly tapered by no more than 25 mcg a week. Slowly decreasing the dose allows the body to adjust to the lower doses of thyroid. Ask the patient to stop decreasing the dose if he or she starts to feel better. Rarely, the optimal dose is missed and only found when decreasing the dose.

If a patient has benefited from HDT and has developed side effects, this is a different situation (see discussion of side effects below).

To Monitor Thyroid Levels or Not Monitor Thyroid Levels, That Is the Question

The question of whether is it important to monitor thyroid levels comes up. Simply put, no! This sounds like heresy, but as explained in chapter 4, it is not. Clinical response is the best way to judge the adequacy of a dose. For a complete discussion, see chapter 13. There are two exceptions. First, if patients were initially hypothyroid or bipolar I, the initial goal should be to bring T3 levels into the high normal range and TSH into the low normal range. The second exception is if you need to check a patient's compliance.

If you do get thyroid blood levels, tell patients what to expect. With T3, usually you can expect that TSH and T4 will be low, and T3 can range from normal to high. If you are using T4, TSH will generally be low, and both T3 and T4 may range from normal to high. It is remarkable, but occasionally, a patient on a very high dose, who has responded well, will have normal T3 levels.

Since we can't rely on blood levels, the best way to monitor adequate levels is the old-fashioned way, through clinical assessment. The bottom line is that if the patient is still having affective symptoms and not experiencing thyrotoxic symptoms, then the dose should be increased. If the patient is receiving benefit from HDT and experiencing thyrotoxic symptoms, then the dose likely should be decreased. There are caveats; see How to Handle Thyroid Side Effects below. If a previous response has decreased, increase the dose. See Thyroid Poop Out: the Need to Increase the Dose over Time below.

How to Handle Thyroid Side Effects

Most of the time, it is easy to distinguish thyrotoxic symptoms from bipolar symptoms. However, it is important to establish whether the patient is indeed experiencing a side effect from the HDT or from another medication, as a result of the underlying affective illness, or from the combination of HDT and another medication—for example, tremors from the combination of lithium and HDT. A tremor when lithium and HDT are used together is common and does not necessarily imply toxicity of either medication. Check if the patient is taking the correct dose of thyroid.

The number of patients who increase or decrease their medication without informing their doctor is surprising.

Thyrotoxic symptoms are: palpitations, increased appetite, anxiety, irritability, tremor, sweating, changes in menstrual patterns, feeling too hot, more frequent bowel movements, fatigue, muscle weakness, difficulty sleeping, skin thinning, fine and brittle hair. Signs of thyrotoxicosis are: tachycardia and weight loss (Monaco, 2012). As you can see, some these symptoms such as irritability, increased appetite, difficulty sleeping, fatigue, irregular menstrual patterns, anxiety, and difficulty sleeping are all common symptoms in the bipolar disorders. These symptoms are likely due to the bipolar—unless they are accompanied by other indications of thyrotoxicity. Most patients welcome weight loss. Weight loss can be a problem if the patient is dropping below normal weight; likewise, an increased appetite is not a problem if it is not accompanied by weight gain. Weight gain from HDT is unlikely, so if it is happening, look for other causes first.

Mild Bone or Joint Pain at Higher Doses

This is usually subtle at the beginning. If the dose is increased, the pain increases. Ask about this side effect from time to time. It may save a patient from getting a costly work-up. Nothing can be done other than slowly reducing the dose until the pain is gone.

Weight Loss

Only a small percentage of patients will experience weight loss, and most will be delighted. This side effect appears to be caused primarily by reduction in appetite, and this alarms some patients. Explain to patients that the HDT has changed the "set point" that their bodies believe is optimum and that their appetite will return when they reach that set point.

Increased Appetite

HDT regularly increases appetite without weight gain.

Palpitations

HDT does have a positive inotropic effect, and patients often notice that their heart is beating stronger. If the palpitations occur with other signs and symptoms of thyrotoxicosis, then a dosage reduction is in order. Otherwise, normalize the experience; palpitations are common with patients suffering anxiety. Palpitations are very common in psychiatric patients and rarely indicate an underling heart problem. Reassure the patient that over time, the palpitations are likely to go away as other bipolar symptoms improve.

If a patient complains of palpitations, the first thing to do is to check his or her pulse. If the pulse is below 100 find out if the patient has a history of palpitations. If so, are the palpitations different or more frequent? If reassurance is not enough, follow the algorithm below labeled **heart rate >100**. Palpitations that happen after the patient has been on the same dose for some time are unlikely to be due to the HDT, unless they are accompanied by other thyrotoxic symptoms.

Heartbeat > 100:

Heart rates > than 100 may predispose patients to develop atrial fibrillation (AF). Make sure that it is truly a resting heart rate. If the patient just ran up five flights of stairs or is upset, this isn't a resting heart rate. Ask how much **caffeine** the patient drank that day. If he or she is vague, ask leading questions such as, "Did you have five or six cups of coffee today?" This gives the patient permission to tell the truth. Ask how big the cups were. Regardless of the amount of caffeine the patient as has, the first thing to do is cut that back or stop caffeine altogether. If the patient elects to stop using caffeine, please remember to warn him or her of caffeine-withdrawal symptoms (see table 1). Withdrawal symptoms should last just a couple of days. Measure the heart rate again on the next visit. If the patient has used caffeine that day and the heart rate continues to be > 100 then choose one or more of the following options:

1. **Measure the heart rate again.** Make sure the patient is calm and relaxed.
2. **Eliminate caffeine.** Caffeine potentiates the effects of HDT on heart rate. You may get a lot of pushback on this. Caffeine is perceived as greatly helping energy and concentration. It is important to point out that HDT can replace caffeine—and usually with better results. Cutting back on caffeine can do much to help anxiety. It is critical for patients to reduce or entirely stop caffeine, as this may reduce the risk of atrial fibrillation. It is important to tell patients this, otherwise they will cheat.
3. **If the heart rate is only rapid in the mornings**, move a portion of the thyroid dose to bedtime. As long as it doesn't interfere with sleep, this is fine.
4. **Consider a low dose of a beta blocker.** Sometimes 10 to 20 mg of propranolol once or twice a day is sufficient. Propranolol XL sometimes will work better for patients who have trouble taking a dose more than twice a day or can get by with a single dose but need coverage longer than regular release propranolol. Atenolol at a dose of 25 mg often works well and covers more of the day than the propranolol does. This is the best option when lowering the thyroid dose would result in the return of unacceptable mood symptoms. If you have exhausted other treatment options, then this is preferable to leaving the patient with unacceptable mood symptoms.
5. **Wait.** If the heart rate between 100 - 110, waiting a week or two may bring the heart rate down.
6. **Cut back on the dose of thyroid.** Generally cutting back by 12.5 to 25 mcg will be enough. Sometimes cutting back 12.5 to 25 mcg every other day will work. If the patient lapses back into a depression, it is time to consider a beta blocker as discussed above.
7. **Side effects and no improvement.** If you are seeing side effects and no improvement, then taper the dose of T3 by 12.5 to 25 mcg weekly. Look for a sweet spot—that is, good control of symptoms without side effects.

Anxiety

Distinguishing between what is related to HDT and/or related to the bipolar disorder can be difficult. Anxiety that increases right after an increase in thyroid dose usually represents a side effect. But don't automatically assume it is the cause. Consider the following:

1. Has there been an actual increase in the amount of anxiety? As patients improve, symptoms that have been present all along are sometimes reported for the first time.
2. Check if the patient is taking the prescribed dose. Sometimes you have to send the patient home to report back the actual amount that he or she has been taking. For example, if the patient is using a pill minder, then have him or her check to see if the correct dose of thyroid was actually laid out.
3. Does the patient regularly cycle in and out of anxious periods? If the anxiety is experienced in the morning after taking the T3 dose, then moving some of the T3 to nighttime can sometimes help. If the patient is cycling over a period of days or weeks, then the anxiety is more likely to be due to diurnal variations of mood symptoms.
4. Is there an external cause for an increase in anxiety? How much caffeine is the patient using? Even if the patient's heart rate is < 100, cutting back on caffeine often takes care of the problem.
5. Is it akathisia caused by a neuroleptic?
6. Check for other signs or symptoms of thyrotoxicity. If the patient is having other symptoms or signs of thyrotoxicity, cut back on the dose.
7. Keep in mind that in some cases, anxiety can be a reemergence of symptoms that represents the need to increase the dose of thyroid.
8. There are two choices: decrease the thyroid dose or, surprisingly, increase it again. The quickest way to find out if the anxiety symptoms are caused by too high a dose of thyroid is to increase the dose yet again. This may not be the wisest way to handle the situation, but it is the quickest and, in some situations, the easiest. Only do this if the patient is willing, there is reason to believe that cutting back on the

dose of thyroid may be a disaster and/or there is reason to believe it is not the HDT that is causing the anxiety. Increasing the thyroid dose by 12.5 mcg of T3 should worsen symptoms if, in fact, the symptoms are caused by too much thyroid hormone.

The other way to ascertain if the dose is too high is to cut back on the dose of T3 by 12.5 to 25 μg every three to seven days until the anxiety is gone. If the anxiety is truly caused by too much T3, then symptoms should improve when the dose has been decreased by 25 to 50 mcg. If anxiety symptoms have not improved, likely the anxiety has a different cause. Discuss what to do if the depression starts to return. Instruct the patient to call. It is likely that increasing the dose of T3 by 12.5 to 25 mcg again will be helpful.
9. Wait. If anxiety symptoms improve, HDT was not the cause.

At least 50% of the time, it just isn't clear why anxiety symptoms have worsened or emerged. The result is that you are forced to cut back on the dose. When decreasing the thyroid dose, it is highly unusual for the symptoms attributed to HDT to worsen or reappear with no improvement in anxiety. This is a clear sign that HDT is not the culprit causing the anxiety.

The most important aspect of this is to watch for a reemergence of mood symptoms that the HDT previously had controlled. If bipolar symptoms reemerge shortly after a decrease in dose, it likely means that HDT was not the source of the problem.

Tremor

How much tremor is too much tremor? Leave that up to the patient's judgment. Sometimes tremors make it impossible to use HDT. Occasionally, patients know the etiology of their tremors. So don't assume; the HDT may not be causing them. Tremors can happen at less than thyrotoxic doses. For example, a tremor when lithium and HDT are combined does not necessarily indicate toxicity from either. Keep in mind that thyroid tremor can involve major muscle groups such as **thigh or calf muscles**. Tremors of the thigh or calf can appear without a hand tremor. Tremors of the thigh will appear when the patient is bending at the knees. Tremors of the calves tend to show up when patients are pushing a car brake. Make sure to reassure patients that the tremor, if it's caused by the HDT, is dose dependent and not permanent. The following questions will be helpful:

1. **Is the tremor new or worse?** Ask if the tremor has been there all along and the patient is just reporting it for the first time.
2. **When did the tremor first appear?** Did it coincide with an increase in thyroid dose or a change in how the patient is taking his or her thyroid dose—for example, moving T4 consumption away from meals to a time when it is better absorbed?
3. Check to see what **nonpsychiatric medications** may be contributing to the tremor.
4. **Check to see what psychiatric medications may be contributing to the tremor**—for example, lithium. The combination of lithium and HDT can be particularly difficult because both may be contributing to the tremor, and it does not necessarily represent toxic levels of either thyroid or lithium. What to do? Decrease the less important of the two. Decreasing the lithium is often the thing to do. Lower doses of lithium sometimes work better, at least in bipolar II or NOS. For bipolar I, a lower lithium dose can work better for depression but may put the patient at risk of mania. But if the lithium was working well, likely the HDT would not have been added in the first place. Normally, the tremor from lithium is dose dependent. This generally is not true with the combination of lithium and HDT. Consideration should be given to tapering and discontinuing the lithium or tapering and stopping HDT, whichever one is deemed less important.
5. Valproic acid and carbamazepine can create a similar situation. Neuroleptics can occasionally cause tremor. Consider a reduction in dose of these medications or thyroid.
6. Does the patient have a family history of tremors? HDT often will worsen these tremors. Occasionally, benign familial

tremor will first appear under HDT, but HDT is not the cause of the tremor.

Tremor treatment:

Decreasing the dose of T3 by 12.5 to 25 mcg can be helpful, usually without the loss of the benefits of HDT. A low-dose beta blocker, for example propranolol 10 mg to 20 mg once or twice a day, can be helpful. Alternatively, beta blockers can be taken PRN. If all else fails, it is up to the patient to choose between the tremor and HDT.

Feeling Too Hot

Establish that the temperature imbalance is not due to a change of weather. Usually the dose will need to be decreased 12.5 to 25 mcg. Caveats: **If the only time a patient has hot flashes is in early morning**, move part of the thyroid dose to bedtime. This likely will make the hot flashes go away.

Perimenopause hot flashes: Occasionally, for women experiencing perimenopause hot flashes, getting too much thyroid can worsen the hot flashes. To discern between natural hot flashes and too much thyroid hormone, ask the patient at the onset of HDT treatment to note any increase in hot flashes. If the hot flashes are new, a reduction in the thyroid dose for a few days with T3 or a week with T4 can make things clear.

Extreme Physical Exhaustion after Hard Physical Workout

It is important to understand that by "extreme," I mean that the physical exhaustion is beyond what the patient normally experiences even with a hard workout. It often necessitates ending a workout early. This is rare and should not be confused with the exhaustion commonly seen with depressions. The exhaustion of depression is usually pervasive or regularly occurs in a particular part of the day. This is part of the bipolar illness and not a side effect. This discussion is limited to **extreme sports or workouts**, such as Ironman competitions, in which competitors swim 2.4 miles, bike 112 miles and run 26.2 miles. The combination of extreme workouts and HDT can strengthen the heart to the point where the heart functions less efficiently. Some extreme athletes will report abnormal exhaustion and are unable to perform at the previous maximal level. It is up to the patient to either cut back on the thyroid dose or cut back on the amount of exercise. This is rare, even among extreme athletes. Clinically, it has not been observed with patients doing normal workouts.

Excruciating Bone or Joint Pain at Low Doses

This is a rare event, occurring in less than 1% of patients and usually appearing at 25 to 50 mcg doses. Most often, it involves the joints of the hands or feet and sometimes the legs. There's nothing to do but stop thyroid entirely and move to a different treatment. Trying smaller doses—even 5 mcg—and slowly increasing the dose is unlikely to overcome the problem.

Hair Loss

Hair loss can be very disturbing to some patients, so it must be taken seriously. Many psychiatric medications seem to be associated with hair loss—for example, valproic acid. Patients with long hair can become the most upset. Hair loss happens in less than 2% of women and never seems to progress to the point that it becomes serious. Women, however, are frightened that it will accelerate. Clinically, it isn't clear that the hair loss is caused by HDT. Drastically cutting back on HDT or even stopping thyroid hormone altogether only helps in 10% of cases and sometimes accelerates the hair loss. With selenium and/or time, the hair loss usually reverses itself. The hair loss may be due to some psychiatric medications that cause selenium depletion. In any event, male pattern baldness is not due to HDT.

This not to say that serious hair loss can't happen. Remember, while it is rare, some women can naturally suffer significant hair loss—even baldness—without exposure to any psychiatric medications. Factors to consider include the following:

1. Hair loss is included in some but not all lists of hyperthyroid symptoms. No research has been located that clearly

identifies HDT as a cause of hair loss. Even the literature for hyperthyroidism shows no systematic evaluations of and for hair loss. Despite the lack of clear research, many books or papers, without providing any references, state that too much thyroid hormone can cause major hair loss. Hypothyroidism can cause severe hair loss. Clinically, hair loss does not appear to be any more prevalent after HDT treatment than before the use of HDT.
2. Check for low testosterone levels both in men and women.
3. Treat with selenium 50 to 200 mcg per day. Often, the selenium in a One A Day vitamin is sufficient. Not all One A Day vitamins contain selenium, so have the patient check the back of the bottle to see if it's present.
4. Reassure the patient that hair loss from medications does not progress to baldness and eventually reverses itself.
5. Discuss whether the patient desires a reduction in the thyroid dose. If you don't, the patient may do it anyway.
6. Consult a dermatologist to look for other causes of hair loss.

Sudden Onset of Thyrotoxic Symptoms

Less than 1% of patients will develop marked thyrotoxic symptoms after experiencing clear benefits from HDT. Why this happens is unknown. This often means that the dose needs to be drastically cut back to 25 mcg of T3 or none at all. Most of these patients will not relapse, despite having experienced great benefits from HDT in the past. Taper the dose of T3 every five days until the symptoms disappear.

Thyroid Poop Out: The Need to Increase the Dose over Time

For unknown reasons, roughly 50% to 60% of patients will need escalations of their thyroid dose over time. Surprisingly, side effects don't increase. The need to increase the dose will be evident if bipolar symptoms reappear or worsen. The emergence of the need for a higher dose is unpredictable and can occur months to years after stability has been achieved. This process of needing to increase the dose can occur a number of times. At doses of approximately

100 to 150 mcg of T3 but occasionally higher, the need for further dose increases no longer occurs. Remind patients of this possibility after the optimal dose is reached and every couple of months thereafter. It is especially important to remind patients of this when you are decreasing the thyroid hormone dose due to side effects, because in the future, their need for thyroid hormone will likely go up. Yesterday's dose that was too high may be today's needed dose. Even if a patient previously experienced side effects at a higher dose, most will experience improvement without side effects at this stage of treatment. It is important to tell the patient that you may be wrong they may need a dose reduction but since they are familiar with what to look for, they can simply deal with it by decreasing the dose. If they are unsure what to do, have them call you.

What to Look For and When to Suspect Poop Out

Any worsening of bipolar symptoms, especially depressive symptoms is sufficient reason by itself. While none of the following clues is required, they reinforce the possibility that poop out is present:

1. Mild side effects have disappeared.
2. Weight gain.
3. Increased sensitivity to cold.
4. Energy problems. Some patients may become lethargic.
5. Thinking/memory problems.
6. Increased vulnerability to stress or report of an increase in stress. At the earliest stages of a relapse, before full symptoms are easily identified, patients often report an increase in stress. Often patients will rationalize this as a result of external events. Evaluate whether the stress reaction is more than what would be expected.
7. The return of boredom. Being bored while one waits at an airport is normal. If one is getting bored with major aspects of one's life that previously were interesting, it is likely the beginning of a relapse.

If it is unclear that a patient's condition has actually worsened, reevaluate in one to three weeks.

How to Handle Interference with HDT Treatment

When other doctors, family, and friends tell the patient to cut back or stop HDT, what should you say to the patient? Remind the patient that you previously discussed that other doctors who are unfamiliar with the scientific literature may oppose HDT out of the mistaken belief that it is causing "hyperthyroidism." Remind the patient that HDT is relatively safe, its effectiveness has been established, and you are following published treatment guidelines. Point out the benefit that the patient has received. Offer to talk directly to the patient's physician or the family member or friend who is advising against HDT. Alternatively, send the letter in the appendix that explains HDT. Give the patient a copy of the letter.

What if the patient wants to stop HDT against medical advice? If the patient is hell-bent on stopping HDT, it is best to do this cooperatively, because the patent likely will stop it anyway. Try to negotiate the longest period of time between dosage reductions. Smaller dosage reductions are best.

Slowly tapering the dose has several benefits:

1. The slow reduction of any psychiatric medication will increase the chance that the taper will be successful. Abruptly stopping or tapering most psychiatric medications too quickly can precipitate a nasty relapse. The relapse may be more difficult to treat than previous relapses have been.

2. The patient's thyroid gland can use the time to "reawaken" and get back into the business of producing its own thyroid hormone. Most patients will accept this.

3. Explain to the patient that because he or she is reducing the dose, he or she will need to be seen more frequently. This, alone, sometimes dissuades patients from an ill-advised course of stopping HDT. Do see the patient more frequently.

4. If there is a relapse because of dosage reduction, reducing the dose slowly may help the patient have a "softer landing." In other words, you will maximize the chance of catching the relapse at an earlier stage, making it easier to facilitate recovery.

If the patient does start to relapse, instruct him or her to increase the dose again.

Unless the patient absolutely insists, never start a taper before a major vacation (either the patient's or yours) or an important holiday or event.

What if the patient has been diagnosed with osteopenia or osteoporosis and told that HDT is the cause?

Osteopenia and osteoporosis occur naturally. Patients who have developed osteopenia or osteoporosis and are treated with appropriate bone-building medications do not progress (and sometimes will improve) even when HDT is continued. Clinically, the rate of women developing osteoporosis has been well within the rates expected from the general population. Of the patients who were on HDT, most either stopped or greatly reduced their thyroid doses. All had to return to HDT because of a severe relapse into depression. Chapter 6 shows the lack of risk of osteoporosis. Here's how to proceed:

1. Explain to the patient that osteopenia or osteoporosis occurs by age sixty in 50% of Caucasian women in the United States. Percentages are lower for other races (Watts et al., 2010). It is not uncommon in women under age fifty.
2. Review the patient's risk factors, which include age, race (either Caucasian or Asian), a family history of osteoporosis, a small body frame, hyperparathyroidism, a history of hyperthyroidism past or present, low calcium intake, low vitamin D levels, past or present eating disorders, previous gastrointestinal surgery, a history of extended use of steroids, early menopause, past or present alcohol abuse or dependence, and past or present tobacco use. One of the biggest risk factors is immobility. For

patients who have spent substantial amounts of time depressed, immobility was usually a part of it. Sleeping 10-14 hours a day, low energy, and low motivation are strong risk factors.
3. Review with the patient that while hyperthyroidism is associated with bone thinning, the scientific literature does not show that HDT is a risk.
4. Reassure the patient that the treatments for low bone mass are effective.
5. Contact the other physician and review all the above. Insist on a full risk-benefit analysis if the other doctor insists on stopping or even decreasing HDT.

What to do if another doctor wants to taper HDT to see if the patient has an underlying hyperthyroidism?

If the patient is not experiencing any thyrotoxic symptoms, then by definition, the patient does not have hyperthyroidism. Measuring antithyroid antibodies can diagnose Graves' disease and lymphocytic thyroiditis without the need to decrease HDT. Other doctors can be insistent on the need to taper HDT, so a frank discussion of the risks and benefits with the patient and the other doctor can be helpful. Most importantly, discuss the risks associated with relapse and the other possible medications.

How to deal with endocrinologists and other physicians:

Expect interference. It is unfortunate that other doctors will interfere with the use of HDT, regardless of how well it works and the lack of side effects. These doctors rarely do a risk-benefit analysis. They usually focus only on the perceived risk of HDT— i.e., the myth that HDT = hyperthyroidism. It is not unusual for endocrinologists or other doctors to instruct patients to stop HDT immediately, regardless of the potential consequences. (See chapters 4, 12, and 13 for more details.) Stopping HDT may precipitate a sudden relapse in the bipolar disorder, usually depression. Suddenly stopping HDT can potentially cause cardiac problems. When it comes to treating psychiatric illnesses and formulating a risk-benefit analysis, the psychiatrist needs to lead the treatment team. (See chapter 15 for more details.) It may help to send the letter (in the appendix) to all doctors involved with the patient. It explains the rationale and the scientific basis for HDT. Giving the patient, the thyroid handout will also help.

What to do if the patient develops atrial fibrillation?

First, don't panic. Some doctors seem to go into near hysteria. While atrial fibrillation (AF) is urgent, it is not an emergency. AF is serious, but as they say, "Take your own pulse first." Many patients go for extended periods of time with AF before it is treated. Some practical steps that other physicians routinely overlook or are not aware of may well stop the AF. They include:

1. Look for other medical causes of AF.
2. If the patient is using any caffeine, simply discontinuing caffeine will sometimes stop AF.
3. Adding a beta blocker may stop the AF.
4. Before discontinuing HDT, a dose reduction may stop the AF. This also avoids the potential cardiac problems that can come from suddenly discontinuing HDT.
5. If all else fails, taper or drastically cut back on the dose of HDT.

Keep in mind that the patient may be angry about getting AF. Whether you believe the HDT was the cause or not, approach the situation with humility. Unless you have discovered the AF, it is likely that some other doctor has placed the blame on the HDT without considering other alternatives. For more in-depth information, see chapters 4, 6, 13, and 14.

Prudent steps include the following:

1. Discuss with the patient that there is a 22.7% lifetime risk for AF, so the HDT may or may not be playing a role (Lloyd-Jones et al., 2004). Review with the patient that while hyperthyroidism is associated with AF, the scientific literature does not show a risk for AF with HDT use.
2. Review the patient's history for known risk factors such as hypertension, valvular disease, cardiomyopathy, diabetes, thyroid disease, previous hypothyroidism or

hyperthyroidism, pneumonia, obesity, sleep apnea, and alcohol and tobacco use. Inflammation is thought to play a role. Always find out how much caffeine the patient is taking in general and how much he or she ingested on the day that the AF developed.
3. Correct for any of the above risk factors that can be controlled. For example, stop caffeine, tobacco, and all alcohol intake, and/or restart sleep apnea treatment. Simply stopping caffeine often will stop AF.
4. Usually, HDT treatment has been stopped before the psychiatrist is made aware of the situation. If the patient is still on HDT, a risk-benefit analysis is in order.
5. The wisest course may be to keep the patient on HDT if the patient has a significant risk of relapse and this risk is higher than of the risk of AF. A discussion with the patient and family may be in order.
    a. Get the patient treated with an appropriate anticlotting agent to prevent a clot from forming on a heart valve.
    b. Review with the patient that there is no literature that suggests that HDT causes any other heart arrhythmias. Even in hyperthyroidism, arrhythmias other than AF are extremely rare.

If the risk-benefit analysis falls on the side of stopping HDT, a quick taper may be needed: 50 mcg initially and then cut the dose by 25 mcg every five to seven days. Monitor the patient before every decrease to assess whether the AF has stopped or bipolar symptoms have returned. Keep in mind that abruptly stopping HDT may carry its own rare cardiac risk. Start a suitable regimen either to prevent the return of bipolar symptoms or to treat symptoms that have returned. Let the patient know that symptoms could return quickly or may be delayed for some time.

Though patients usually won't want to talk about the possible return to HDT at this time, it is important to plant the seed that many patients can and do safely return to HDT after an AF is controlled. This is important. If the patient's mood drops substantially, just the idea that he or she can safely return to HDT may prevent a suicide.

On subsequent meetings, if HDT has been stopped:

1. Review any of the points above that may need to be reinforced.
2. As time goes by and subsequent treatments fail, the patient may need to return to HDT. Reassure the patient that usually we are able to return to HDT without the reoccurrence of AF, and the risks can be minimized if closely monitored.

Clinically, every patient who stopped HDT saw the AF spontaneously stop. The one patient whose risk-benefit analysis compelled the need to continue HDT is alive and well after eight years of AF. She is now ninety-five years old. For more details about HDT and AF experiences, see chapter 7.

Chapter 3: Important Definitions

To practice evidence-based medicine, one must first start with evidenced-based definitions.

—Tammas Kelly, MD

Case report: Jenny was a 32-year-old female who, despite many trials of medications including lithium, valproic acid, carbamazepine, quetiapine, and many others, struggled with bipolar I depression. She would often spend 16 hours a day in bed. She became euthymic with HDT. She had no side effects from her 75 mcg of T3. Her primary-care physician became alarmed at her low TSH and wanted her to cut back. The primary-care physician labeled that condition iatrogenic hyperthyroidism. She had no signs of thyrotoxicosis. T3 and T4 levels were eventually obtained and were in the upper limit of normal.

HDT and Thyroid Augmentation

The definition of high-dose thyroid (HDT) is historically based. HDT therapy with T3 is defined as doses of > 50 mcg (Kelly and Lieberman, 2009). HDT for T4 is 200 mcg and above (Bauer et al., 2003). The term "augmentation" has been consistently used in the psychiatric literature for T3 doses ≤ 50 mcg. It is important to note that the definition of HDT when used in psychiatry does not rely on blood levels. The reasons are explained in chapter 4. Endocrinologists use different terms to refer to HDT. This book will use psychiatric terminology.

Typically, HDT suppresses TSH. A low TSH—even a very low TSH—does not automatically mean that T3 or T4 levels are elevated. Not infrequently, patients treated with HDT can have super depressed TSH, yet still have normal levels of T3. Most often with T3 HDT, T4 will be low and T3 will be high. This book will present research that shows why thyroid blood levels are irrelevant for bipolar individuals. Bipolar patients may, in fact, be suffering from cellular hypothyroidism regardless of serum thyroid levels. See chapter 13.

Definitions of Hyperthyroidism and Thyrotoxicosis

It is critically important to distinguish the fundamental differences between hyperthyroidism and high circulating levels of thyroid hormone caused by thyroid medication. Although the two are often erroneously equated, the latter does not meet the formal definition of hyperthyroidism regardless of how high the blood levels are. These differences are explored in more detail below and will become critically important to understanding the differences in the risks of hyperthyroidism and HDT All definitions of hyperthyroidism and thyrotoxicosis are similar to the definitions used by the joint task force of the American Thyroid Association and the American Association of Clinical Endocrinologists' management guidelines on hyperthyroidism treatment.

Hyperthyroidism is defined as the overproduction of endogenous thyroid hormone with accompanying signs and symptoms of thyrotoxicosis. **Thyrotoxicosis is defined** as the presence of signs and symptoms of high circulating levels of thyroid hormone. Both definitions require confirmation by laboratory studies of high levels of thyroid hormone. Hyperthyroidism is a subtype of thyrotoxicosis. Subclinical hyperthyroidism is considered a mild form of hyperthyroidism and defined by TSH levels below normal, with normal T3 and T4 levels. It may or may not be accompanied by thyrotoxic symptoms (Bahn et al., 2011), (Mansourian, 2010), (Trzepacz et al., 1989), (Mandel, 2011). The proper way to refer to high circulating levels of thyroid hormone due to taking external thyroid hormone in the absence of thyrotoxic symptoms is **hypertyrosinemia** (Bauer et al., 2003).

Despite these definitions, endocrinologists and many other medical personnel consider that use of HDT causes hyperthyroidism, usually based on low TSH. This is despite the absence of signs and symptoms of thyrotoxicity. See chapters 4, 13, and 14.

Thyroid Storm

The only reason to discuss thyroid storm is that other doctors will worry about the possibility or mistakenly assert that a patient is suffering from thyroid storm. Thyroid storm is a rare, potentially life-threatening event that stems from a massive release of thyroid hormone from the thyroid gland. The thyroid gland can store a week's worth of thyroid hormone. Most cases of thyroid storm are associated with some surgical manipulation of the thyroid gland. There has never been a reported case of thyroid storm with HDT. In fact, since HDT leads to a decrease of thyroid hormone content within the thyroid gland, HDT may decrease the risk for thyroid storm. The decrease of thyroid content would likely be dependent on the suppression of TSH.

For the purposes of this book, **clinical impression** is defined as a preliminary observation based on fewer than 10 patients. Clinical impressions are, of course, are always suspect, and they represent the very lowest rung of scientific evidence. Clinical impressions are not wholly without merit, however. They are particularly important in rare phenomena—for example, treating the psychiatric problems associated with Huntington's chorea, where there is a complete lack of research on how to treat psychiatric aspects of Huntington's. Treatment decisions based on clinical impressions should be limited to situations where absolutely all valid treatments have failed. In other words, they should be extremely rare. Clinical impressions should be considered an invitation for more careful observation. Where would we be today if John Cade's experience with lithium treatment of 10 manic patients had been dismissed as a "clinical impression"?

Clinical observation, abbreviated in this book as "clinical" or "clinically," are conclusions based at least on the experiences and observations of >100 patients. In the case of this book, my clinical observations are based on experiences of over 1500 trials of thyroid treatment over the years. Most but not all trials of thyroid hormone were with high doses. To be certain, not all trials were successful. I have published a number of studies based on the systematic evaluation of my observations with HDT and other medications. (Kelly, 2008; Kelly et al., 2013; Kelly and Lieberman, 2009; Kelly and Lieberman, 2017)

Chapter 4: Why HDT Isn't Hyperthyroidism

The most exciting phrase to hear in science, the one that heralds new discoveries, is not 'Eureka!' but 'That's funny...'
–Isaac Asimov

Summary: This chapter reviews the more-than-ample evidence that HDT does not equate with hyperthyroidism.

This book came about from a "that's funny" experience. When I was researching the risk of HDT, I noticed a large discrepancy between the risk as stated in the endocrine literature and the risk that the literature actually shows for HDT. Moreover, there was an even larger discrepancy between the medical sequela of hyperthyroidism and what the literature shows the risk of HDT to be. Mark Twain stated, "Education consists mainly in what we have unlearned." Prepare yourself to unlearn something.

Evidence that HDT and Hyperthyroidism Are Not the Same

When using T3 HDT, most patients' TSH levels drop below normal, with low T4 levels. T3 levels range from normal to extremely high. Physicians who are not familiar with HDT literature showing the safety of HDT are extremely uncomfortable with this, regardless of the benefits of HDT. There is some rather remarkable experimental evidence that HDT in affective disorders is fundamentally different than hyperthyroidism. As illustrated in chapters 6 and 7, HDT does not pose a risk for osteoporosis, increase cardiac problems, or increase mortality. In other words, HDT in affective disorders has some remarkably positive effects and is fundamentally different from hyperthyroidism.

HDT Is Well Tolerated

Clinically, it is not unusual to find patients on a dose of 200 mcg of T3 with no side effects and showing great improvement (if not frank euthymia) without side effects. Multiple studies have shown how well patients with an affective disease tolerate HDT treatment (Bauer et al., 2003; Bauer et al., 2002; Bauer et al., 2015; Bauer et al., 2005; Bauer and Whybrow, 2001; Bauer and Whybrow, 1990; Kelly and Lieberman, 2009; Ricken et al., 2012a). Moreover, patients with affective disorders demonstrate a fundamentally different response to HDT therapy compared with nonaffectively ill individuals. HDT is far better tolerated. There is a remarkable study that directly compared the effects of HDT treatment in a group of refractory depressed patients (bipolar and major depression) with a matched control group of nonaffectively ill, normal volunteers. How normal can you be to volunteer for this type of research is an open question, but at least the volunteers were not psychiatrically ill, nor did they have any thyroid problems. Both groups started with a dose of 100 mcg/d of T4 and increased it by 100 mcg/d each week until the dose of 500 mcg/d was achieved. This dose was maintained for an additional four weeks. Thyrotoxic symptoms caused 38% of the control group to discontinue T4, many before the full dose was reached. None of the patients in the T4 augmentation group discontinued treatment. Patients in the control and treatment groups had similar average thyroid levels prior to HDT treatment. At the end of the study, TSH levels were equally suppressed. The affectively ill group had significantly lower T3 and T4 levels compared with the control group. In the group with refractory depression, average HAM-D scores decreased from 27.0 to 10.7 compared with an increase of HAM-D scores from 0.9 to 5.2 in the control group (Bauer et al., 2002).*

*The very first time I reviewed this study and every subsequent time I reviewed it, I thought, "These normal volunteers had to have been the author and the author's friends and colleagues around the clinic." I caught up with first author Michael Bauer at the 2016 International Society for Bipolar Disorders conference in Amsterdam. Sure enough, he confirmed my suspicion. He told me that they were all intensely uncomfortable and sweating when taking 500 mcg of T4. This is not to imply that patients with bipolar disorders are immune from thyrotoxic symptoms; it suggests only that thyrotoxic symptoms don't necessarily occur even with high blood levels of thyroid. In the normal routine of HDT treatment, if the dose is raised high enough, symptoms can develop, and the dose is decreased.

By contrast, thyroid cancer survivors often do not tolerate HDT well. In thyroid cancer survivors, too high a thyroid level can impair psychological, social, and physical functioning, especially with very low TSH ranges (Biondi and Kahaly, 2010). The tolerance of HDT may well be an important indication of why HDT works. Please see chapters 5 and 13.

HDT Normalizes Brain Physiology

Is HDT doing more than just treating symptoms? There is good evidence that HDT has positive physiologic effects on the bipolar brain. In fact, a number of studies show that HDT has positive effects on neurophysiology. The most eloquent evidence comes from two [F-18]-2-fluorodeoxyglucose positron emission tomography (FDG-PET) studies that show remarkable changes in the brain when HDT is added. A priori, one would expect that extra thyroid hormone would increase brain metabolism, yet the opposite is true. In essence, HDT normalizes the brains of bipolar individuals.

The first FDG-PET study showed normalization of a hypermetabolic state in the prefrontal and limbic areas of the brains of HDT-treated subjects. Ten women suffering from refractory bipolar depression were compared with a matched, healthy control group. When compared with healthy controls, FDG-PET scans showed women with bipolar disorders to have increased activity in the right subgenual cingulate cortex, left thalamus, medial temporal lobe (right amygdala, right hippocampus), right ventral striatum, and cerebellar vermis. The bipolar group was started on 100 mcg/d of T4, added to the existing medications, and increased to 400 mcg/d by the third week. Seven women became euthymic, and three showed improvement. None of the patients dropped out due to side effects. At the end of seven weeks, FDG-PET scans showed decreased brain activity that was indistinguishable from normal brain activity in the right subgenual cingulate cortex, left thalamus, right amygdala, right hippocampus, right dorsal and ventral striatum, and cerebellar vermis. The decrease in depressive symptoms correlated with decreased activity in the left thalamus, left amygdala, left hippocampus, and left ventral striatum (Bauer et al., 2005).

The second FDG-PET study was the first randomized, double-blind, placebo-controlled study showing the efficacy of

HDT. Imaging showed a "significant decrease in regional activity in the left thalamus, right amygdala, right hippocampus, left ventral striatum, and the right dorsal striatum. Decreases in the left thalamus, left dorsal striatum and the subgenual cingulate were correlated with a reduction in depression scores." The treatment group consisted of 25 depressed individuals (15 with bipolar I and 10 with bipolar II) taking 300 mg of T4 (Bauer et al., 2015).

These studies show that HDT significantly normalizes neurophysiology that is directly correlated with decreases in bipolar symptoms.

What Does Cause the Damage in Hyperthyroidism: the Role of Thyroid Antibodies

Why does hyperthyroidism cause osteoporosis and heart problems while HDT treatment does not? Graves' disease and toxic multinodular goiter account for 80% of hyperthyroidism in areas where iodine is readily available in the diet. Both toxic multinodular goiter and Graves' disease have significant autoimmune components. Graves' disease is an autoimmune disease caused by TSH receptor (TSHr) antibodies that mimic the thyroid-stimulating properties of TSH (Biondi and Kahaly, 2010). These TSHr antibodies stimulate TSH receptors, causing the high circulating levels of thyroid hormone in the absence of TSH (Bahn et al., 2011). The TSHr antibody has previously been referred to as the "long acting thyroid stimulator." Autoimmune antibodies are now accepted as the cause of exophthalmos (Wall and Lahooti, 2010) and Graves' dermopathy, also known as pretibial myxoedema (Topliss and Eastman, 2004). There is growing evidence that the osteoporosis associated with hyperthyroidism is mediated by TSHr antibodies (Schett and David, 2010). TSH receptors were identified in cardiac tissue as far back as 1995 (Drvota et al., 1995).

High Bone-Turnover Markers

On the face of it, it would seem that high bone-turnover markers would be a proxy for bone loss. In fact, high bone-turnover markers are offered as "proof" that HDT is a risk factor for osteoporosis. Yet the link between decreasing bone mass and high bone-turnover markers is a correlation. Cause and effect has never definitively been established. There is a study that shows high circulating levels of thyroid hormone that generate high bone-turnover markers do not result in bone loss. Further, the study shows that in previously hyperthyroid individuals, bone loss can occur after thyroid hormone levels are normalized. The study by Balaya and associates, which is discussed in chapter 6, of the effects of high circulating levels of thyroid hormone offers evidence that high bone-turnover markers do not automatically cause bone loss per se. Further, it shows that hyperthyroidism can cause a decrease in bone mass even when thyroid levels are normal. This is the only study that directly examines the effects of high bone-turnover markers, HDT, and the effects of hyperthyroidism. The authors compared four groups of postmenopausal women: a group of patients treated with HDT to suppress reoccurrence of thyroid cancer, a normal control group (without any thyroid disturbances or cancer), a group of patients with Graves' hyperthyroidism, and a group with toxic multinodular goiter hyperthyroidism. Both hyperthyroid groups had received antithyroid treatments for an average of three years prior to the start of the study that resulted in normal T3 and T4 levels for at least six months prior to the start of the study. Bone mass densities were evaluated at the beginning of the study and again after an average of three years of treatment. The group that suffered from thyroid cancer was treated with T4 HDT for at least three years, some longer. It is important to note that the HDT group was the only group to have high circulating thyroid levels during the study. All three of the treatment groups had elevated bone-turnover markers, indicating an increase in osteoblast activity and a decrease in osteoclast activity. Yet despite the high bone-turnover markers, the HDT-thyroid cancer group did not show a decrease in bone mass. Both hyperthyroid groups, despite having normal levels of circulating thyroid, demonstrated significant bone loss (Belaya et al., 2007).

    This study points out two of the critical points that show that HDT is fundamentally different than hyperthyroidism.

    The thyroid cancer group, which was the only group that had high circulating levels of thyroid hormone during the study, had no significant loss of bone mass despite having high bone-turnover markers.

Elevated bone-turnover markers were present in hyperthyroid patients, even though they had normal thyroid levels. This, in turn, points to the facts that hyperthyroidism continues to be a risk factor for osteoporosis even after thyroid levels have been normalized and that the process of reduced BMD is mediated by factors other than high circulating levels of thyroid hormone—for example, TSH receptor antibodies affecting TSH receptors on bones.

Subclinical Hyperthyroidism

The early subclinical hyperthyroidism research (TSH levels below normal, normal T3 and T4 levels) was mixed. Some of the research showed an increase in morbidity and mortality, and some did not. It was not until patients using HDT to prevent the recurrence of thyroid cancer were excluded from the research that subclinical hyperthyroidism consistently showed morbidity and mortality similar to but less than frank hyperthyroidism. This is significant because patients with subclinical hyperthyroidism have normal T3 and T4 levels, yet they are still seeing sequela of hyperthyroidism. Why doesn't HDT cause the same sequela as hyperthyroidism does?

Chapter 5: Evidence That HDT Works and Works Well

Many errors, of a truth, consist merely in the application of the wrong names of things.

−Spinoza

In short: There is ample evidence that HDT works and works well. Clinically, most patients benefit, many becoming euthymic. The evidence indicates that the response to HDT is on par and perhaps better than many medications accepted for treatment of bipolar depression. HDT works far better than antidepressants do for patients with bipolar and without risk of destabilization. There is no evidence to indicate that HDT would work as a sole medication.

The use of thyroid hormone in psychiatry dates back at least as far as 1904, when desiccated sheep thyroid was used to treat "myxedema madness" or severe hypothyroidism (Keaepelin, 1902). HDT first showed success for "cyclic disorders of periodic catatonia" in the 1930s. At that time, hypermetabolic doses of desiccated sheep thyroid were employed (Bauer and Whybrow, 1990). Perhaps one of the reasons that HDT has not been more widely accepted is that there is no drug company to champion it and no drug reps to promote its use.

A great number of published case series, both small and large, indicate the benefit of HDT. This chapter focuses primarily on the treatment of the bipolar disorders and shows that HDT is both efficacious and effective. All of the modern HDT bipolar studies are examined. Roughly speaking, *efficacious* means that a medicine does work, and *effective* reflects how well a medication can work. Randomized, double-blind, placebo-controlled studies are the primary means by which we show that a medication is efficacious. However, randomized, double-blind, placebo-controlled studies give little indication of how well it might work. It isn't until medication is in widespread use that we actually start to understand how effective a medication can be. Large case series and/or numerous small case series can be more helpful in evaluating if a treatment is effective, particularly when the studies are of longer duration than seen in double-blind, placebo-controlled studies. Factors that are important in determining the effectiveness of a medication are cost, the frequency and seriousness of side effects, long-term risks, patient acceptance, patient compliance, and the degree of improvement. Even factors as mundane as how many times a day a medication must be taken are an important determinate of how effective a medication can be.

Except for one failed study discussed below, every study of HDT indicates that it is effective and efficacious for the treatment of the bipolar disorders. This does not imply that HDT is effective for every single patient, nor does it work as a sole treatment for the bipolar disorders. It is widely helpful.

High Normal Thyroid Levels Are Good News (No Thyroid Augmentation or HDT Involved)

At least five studies show that the higher a patient's natural thyroid level is, the better the outcome for bipolar disorders. None of these studies involved extra thyroid medications. In a study performed by Cole and associates at the University of Pittsburg, 65 bipolar I depressed patients were treated with various medications to stabilize moods. The lower the pretreatment TSH and the higher the free thyroxine index, the faster the remission rate (Cole et al., 2002). Chakrabarti reports in his review of thyroid functions and bipolar disorders two studies that show a similar relationship between low T3 and T4 levels and poor short-term outcome of the mania (Chakrabarti, 2011). Additionally, Frye and associates reported that a lower mean level of free T4 was associated with more affective episodes and greater severity of depression during the first year of lithium treatment (Frye et al., 1999). Similar findings have been reported in unipolar depression (Frye et al., 1999; Prange Jr et al., 1990).

Case Series Evidence

The largest psychiatric study of HDT for the treatment of the bipolar disorders was published in 2009 by this author. It is perhaps the largest and longest bipolar II/NOS study to date. This study was used as the only reference for inclusion of HDT in the Canadian Network for Mood and Anxiety Treatments (CANMAT) and International Society for Bipolar Disorders (ISBD) collaborative update of CANMAT guidelines for the management of patients with bipolar disorder: update 2013 (Yatham et al., 2013). When evaluating this study, keep in mind that 95% of these patients would normally be excluded from a randomized, placebo-controlled study because they have failed more than five medications. A total of 159 patients, 125 bipolar II and 34 NOS, were treated for mean of 20.3 months. This was a retrospective chart review. T3 was added to existing medications. Prior to starting T3, patients had failed to stabilize after an average 14 trials of other medications. Efficacy was assessed with the Clinical Global Impression-Improvement (CGI-I) score, which is a seven-point scale ranging from one (very much improved) to seven (very much worse). The criteria for remission was higher than what is normally required in studies, that is, a GAF Score of 80 or more for at least two follow-up appointments, usually within six weeks. Over 82% of bipolar II patients saw significant improvement, mean CGI-I of 1.9, and 84% of bipolar NOS patients showed a significant improvement, mean CGI-I of 1.8. CGI scores of 1.8–1.9 are on par with or better than most treatments. Full remission was achieved in 32% of bipolar II and 38% of bipolar NOS patients. All of the patients had been almost continuously ill for a minimum of two years, many for more than five years, making spontaneous improvement unlikely. The average dose of T3 was 90 mcg. HDT was well tolerated by patients; the vast majority experienced no side effects. Side effects caused 10% of patients to discontinue HDT. These dropouts were not included in the above numbers. No patients became hypomanic or manic during treatment and less than 2% became more depressed. The worsening depression was likely due to overwhelming stress or a natural worsening of the depression. In any event, the side effects experienced by patients were minimal and easily reversed with dosage reduction. Despite this study being the largest HDT study in psychiatry, there are more eloquent and important HDT studies (discussed below).

Since the publication of the study, clinical observations all mirror the outcome of the study. There are two exceptions: first, on rare occasions a few patients have reported a limited number of mild hypomanic symptoms lasting less than a week. These either spontaneously improved without intervention or improved with dose reduction. This is similar to the occasional hypomanic symptoms seen with low-dose lamotrigine, low-dose carbamazepine, low-dose valproic acid, and low-dose aripiprazole. The second exception is that over time, the average dose of T3 or T4 needed to maintain patients has increased. See chapter 12.

Over 500 patients have been treated with HDT at the Depression & Bipolar Clinic of Colorado. Clinically, most patients show great improvement, and at least 25% become long-term euthymic. This is echoed in the literature, which shows that HDT has helped a high percentage of individuals reach long-term euthymia and be more functional than they would otherwise. In other words, it is an essential component in many patients' treatment. This is not to say that HDT is a panacea; other bipolar medications are needed.

Over the years, observations have been made on countless patients who either stop or reduce their doses of T3 AMA. The vast majority relapse, some immediately. Some relapse months later. Returning to the previous T3 dose usually restores the previous gains. Interestingly, a small minority did not relapse when stopping T3, even though T3 was of significant benefit when it was initiated. A later relapse cannot be ruled out.

A 2005 study by Bauer and associates looked at T4 in bipolar disorders, nine with bipolar I and one with bipolar II. This research was primarily designed to study the effects of HDT on brain function using FDG-PET. These effects are discussed at the end of the chapter. All patients were female. Seven patients achieved remission, and three showed a partial response (Bauer et al., 2005).

Randomized, Double-Blind, Placebo-Controlled Studies of HDT for Bipolar Disorders

There have been two randomized, double-blind, placebo-controlled studies of HDT for the treatment of the bipolar disorders. Both groups of researchers involved in these studies deserve much credit. Double-blind, placebo controlled studies are extraordinarily difficult to perform—more so without the deep pockets of a drug company.

The first study consisted of 35 patients with bipolar I and 27 patients with bipolar II. Patients were randomized to T4 add-on therapy or placebo. T4 was started at 100 mcg/d for the first week, 200 mcg/d for the second week, and 300 mcg/d thereafter. Prior to starting T4, all patients from both the control group and the treatment groups had normal TSH, T4, and T3 levels. Outcome was measured at six weeks. At the end of the study, the treatment group showed, as would be expected, significantly low TSH and significantly high T3 and T4. The treatment response was numerically superior but failed to reach statistical improvement. This was primarily due to a high placebo response. An ad hoc analysis did show significant improvement with female patients. One patient dropped out due to mania, one patient dropped out due to thyrotoxic symptoms, and one patient dropped out due to developing a rash with fever (Stamm et al., 2014). In the T3 study discussed above (Kelly and Lieberman, 2009), response and remission rates were the same for men and women. It is possible that the patient who dropped out due to thyrotoxic symptoms might have responded a lower dose without thyrotoxic symptoms.

The important HDT treatment study was performed by Dr. Bauer and associates. This study is important both because it was a FDG-PET imaging study and because it was the first randomized, double-blind, placebo-controlled study that showed HDT efficacy. It consisted of 25 patients suffering from a refractory bipolar disorder, 15 with bipolar II and 10 with bipolar I. Patients were randomized to T4 add on therapy or placebo. T4 was started at 100 mcg/d for the first week, 200 mcg/d for the second week, and 300 mcg/d thereafter. Prior to starting T4, all patients from both groups had normal TSH, T4, and T3 levels. At the end of six weeks, the group receiving 300 mcg of T4 had the following mean levels that showed significantly lower TSH and significantly higher T3 and T4 than the control group. There was no significant change in blood pressure, heart rate, or weight in either group. The mean starting HAMD was 21.7 for the T4 group and 20.3 for the control group. At the end of six weeks, the mean HAMD was 12.6 for the T4 group, and the control group was 16.3. Even though the HAMD difference was small, this was statistically significant. This study also demonstrated the FDG-PET changes in brain functions as a result of HDT (Bauer et al., 2015). See end of the chapter for neuroimaging results. A criticism of this study is the inclusion of a patient taking carbamazepine. Carbamazepine can greatly reduce thyroid blood levels of oral thyroid hormones due to first-pass effects. It would be interesting if this patient showed a response.

Criticism and Applause of Both Double-Blind, Placebo-Controlled Studies

Both of the double-blind, placebo-controlled studies used conservative doses of T4. Prior research has used 400 or 500 mcg without problems. A T4 dose of 300 mcg is equivalent to a dose of T3 of around 75 mcg. Clinical experience suggests that most patients usually start to respond when T3 reaches 75 to 125 mcg. Some patients need even higher doses before showing response. Even more curious are the designs of the studies. T4 has a half-life of seven days, which means that steady-state levels could not be achieved until five weeks after final dosage adjustment. The dose of T4 did not reach the dose of 300 mcg until the third week, and the study was completed at six weeks. It is possible that the conservative dosing and the short study time contributed to the failure of the first study and limited the results of the second.

Thyroid Augmentation

In the literature, thyroid augmentation is defined as a dose of T3 from 25 to 50 mcg (Kelly and Lieberman, 2009) or a dose of T4 of 200 mcg or less (Bauer et al., 2003). Thyroid augmentation can be useful either for accelerating improvement or as maintenance medication. Bauer and Whybrow reviewed seven randomized, double-blind, placebo-controlled studies. T3 augmentation did accelerate improvement of major depression or bipolar depression in five of the seven studies. (Bauer and Whybrow, 2001). In the STAR*D major depression trials, T3 was numerically superior to lithium, but this did not reach statistical difference. However, T3 was far better tolerated (Sinyor et al., 2010).

Michel Bauer and Associates' Excellent Review Article on HDT

This is an older review, and it was instrumental to using HDT. Bauer and associates looked at augmentation of unipolar depression, treatment of bipolar disorder, and maintenance of euthymia in bipolar disorder (Bauer et al., 2003). It is worth reading. The highlights are summarized as follows:

Augmentation, four unipolar studies

In unipolar depression, 37.5 mcg of T3 showed nine out of seventeen responders and worked better than 150 mcg of T4 with four out of twenty-one responders. In a treatment-resistant study of major depression, eight patients responded, two were partial responders, and seven had no response with T4, mean dose 482, range 300–600. In another study of largely unipolar patients, 200 mcg of T4 worked better than lithium. In a study of nine chronically depressed patients, there was a 55% response rate to T4, dose range 150–300 mcg.

HDT study results of bipolar disorders

In the first study, none of the men showed improvement (n=2). Eight women stopped rapid cycling, with three of the eight women showing partial response with T4 at 240–500 mcg. The time frame was nine months to nine years. In the second study, a group of 11 patients, most with hypothyroidism, were treated with T4, dose range 150–400 mcg. This resulted in nine responders, one partial responder, and one with no response. Patients were treated for four to five months. In the third study, six patients suffering a bipolar disorder were treated with T4 ranging from 50–325 mcg for five weeks to three years. Of the six, two patients were responders, two had partial response, and two showed no response. In the fourth study, 20 patients were treated with a mean of 377.5 mcg (range 200–600). There was a significant decrease in episodes, and 52% were judged to be very much improved, and 19% were much improved. Bauer commented that HDT was remarkably well tolerated. Dr. Bauer also commented that T4 is safe to use and causes few side effects (see T3 vs. T4, chapter 11).

HDT for maintenance of euthymia in bipolar disorders, four studies

In three studies totaling 57 patients, 70% were judged to be responders, 22% were judged to be partial responders, and, 18% showed no response. The doses used were highly variable, ranging from 50 to 500 mcg. In the fourth study of 20 patients that used doses of T4 ranging from 200 to 600 mcg, mean of 377 mcg, 52% were judged to be very much improved, and 19% of patients were judged to be much improved (Bauer et al., 2003).

ECT and T3

In multiple animal-model studies, T3 has been shown to decrease neurocognitive side effects and depression. Likewise, multiple human studies have shown that T3 augmentation increases the efficacy of ECT and decreases the neurocognitive side effects. One double-blind study showed that T3 augmentation decreased the number of ECT treatments by 25% (Prange Jr et al., 1990).

Rapid Cycling

Hypothyroidism and low normal thyroid levels have been associated with rapid cycling (Bauer and Whybrow, 1990; Chakrabarti, 2011). While HDT has shown some promise for rapid cycling, not all research has agreed. The research into rapid cycling has been plagued by inadequate doses of HDT and/or inadequate treatment with other medications. In an open-label trial, 10 of 11 rapid-cycling bipolar patients (five with bipolar I and six with bipolar II) with depression at baseline, and five of seven patients with mania at baseline responded to T4, range 150–400 mcg, added to their mood-stabilizing treatment regimens (Bauer and Whybrow, 1990). Side effects were minimal. Clinical response of patients was independent of initial thyroid status. Functionality also improved for most of the 10 patients who showed symptom improvement. Four of the 10 patients entered into an add-on, blinded, placebo crossover study. The other six refused, not wishing to jeopardize the improvement they experienced with HDT. Three of the four patients experienced a return of rapid cycling or a severe relapse after their T4 dose was either stopped or greatly reduced.

HDT is well tolerated, efficacious, and effective both in the short run and in the long run. Not being afraid to increase the dose is important. As long as patients are not experiencing side effects, there is no reason not to increase the dose. HDT, like every medication, is not a panacea but it does work for around 70 to 80% of patients. Most studies comment that HDT was well tolerated, and as we will see in the following chapters, it is as safe as or safer than many of the alternative medications.

One of the most important aspects of HDT is that it often restores functioning, particularly cognitive functioning. This makes it unique among psychiatric medications. Most psychiatric medications used to treat the bipolar disorders can lower functioning—for example, sedation, cognitive dulling, or concentration problems. Also, a unique aspect of HDT, weight loss or gain, is not a significant problem; unfortunately, only a small percentage of overweight or obese patients will experience the profound weight loss. More about weight loss and cognitive functioning in chapter 13.

Normalizing Brain Functioning

Evidence That HDT and Hyperthyroidism Are Not the Same

When using T3 HDT, most patients' TSH levels drop below normal with low T4 levels. T3 levels range from normal to extremely high. Physicians not familiar with HDT literature showing the safety of HDT may be uncomfortable, regardless of the benefits of HDT. There is some rather remarkable experimental evidence that HDT in affective disorders is fundamentally different than hyperthyroidism. As will be illustrated in chapters 5 and 6, HDT does not pose a risk for osteoporosis, nor does it increase cardiac problems or increase mortality. In other words, HDT for affective disorders has some remarkably positive effects and is fundamentally different from hyperthyroidism.

Chapter 6: The Myth That HDT Causes Osteoporosis

There are three kinds of lies: lies, damned lies, and statistics.

–Mark Twain

The short version: There is substantial evidence that HDT is not a risk factor for bone loss. The evidence used to assert that HDT is a risk factor fails to hold up scientifically.

Case study: HJ was a 62 year-old Hispanic male suffering from bipolar II. In his own words, "I drank like a fish," and suffered frequent blackouts for over 20 years. He also "smoked like a dragon," averaging two or more packs of cigarettes a day for more than thirty 30 years. The last 20 years, he suffered from continuous depression, cycling between mild and severe depression. His last clear hypomanic episode was more than 30 years ago. In mild depression, he had minimal physical activity. In his severe depression, he slept 12 to 14 hours a day and spent another two to four hours a day on the couch. In other words, there was almost no activity. He had seen several psychiatrists in the past who treated him primarily with Depakote and antidepressants with minimal success. Eventually, he was tried on a combination of lamotrigine, low-dose oxcarbazepine, and low-dose aripiprazole. He showed some improvement, yet he still cycled between mild and moderate depression. High-dose thyroid was started, and he responded well to 100 mcg. He spontaneously stopped drinking and eventually even managed to quit smoking. After 18 months of treatment with HDT, he was seen by an internist who was alarmed by his low TSH and ordered a bone scan that showed osteopenia. The internist attributed his osteopenia to the HDT and recommended that he stop all thyroid treatment. His depression was severe enough that he chose to continue on HDT. Two years later, a bone scan showed that the osteopenia had resolved. He received no treatment for the osteopenia.

Discussion of case: The internist, as will be shown in this chapter, incorrectly placed the blame on the HDT, overlooking the significant contribution of his bone loss from marked inactivity, alcohol, cigarettes, antidepressants, and Depakote, which are all known risk factors for osteoporosis.

This chapter expands on the published review: a favorable risk-benefit analysis of high dose thyroid for treatment of bipolar disorders with regard to osteoporosis (Kelly, 2014, 2015). It also corrects some errors made in the review.

As we saw in the chapters 3, 4, and 5, the myth that HDT causes osteoporosis stems from the mistaken belief that HDT causes "iatrogenic hyperthyroidism." The understanding that hyperthyroidism is a possible immune disease allows us to reexamine and limit our review to just studies that use HDT. This present chapter will be confined to discussing the scientific literature regarding the use of HDT and the risk of osteoporosis. This myth is pervasive throughout the medical literature. This necessitates an analysis of why endocrinology equates HDT with hyperthyroidism. At first glance, this chapter and the next may seem to be tedious. At second glance, they *are* tedious, but who ever said that science was easy? This is necessary to fully grasp the evidence base to understand why HDT is not a risk for decreasing bone mass. Since it is likely that you will have to discuss this with your medical colleagues until HDT is more widely accepted, it is best to be armed with full knowledge and full understanding.

When considering the literature discussed below, it is important to keep in mind the contrast of HDT and hyperthyroidism. There is no doubt that hyperthyroidism is a major risk factor for osteoporosis, with most studies reporting a 12–20% reduction of bone mass (Lakatos 2003).

The evidence that high circulating levels of thyroid hormone from exogenous sources does not cause a significant decrease in bone mass comes from two sources. First, HDT is routinely used to prevent the return of thyroid cancer. There are a large number of studies looking at the potential risks (Cooper et al., 2009; Kelly, 2016; Perros et al., 2014). The second source is a smaller body of studies of HDT used to treat the bipolar disorders.

When evaluating the safety of HDT, it is critically important to consider only the relevant data. In other words, only studies that examine high circulating levels of thyroid hormone caused by the external use of thyroid hormone should be considered. As we saw in chapter 5, hyperthyroidism, subclinical hyperthyroidism, and hypothyroidism are known risk factors for osteoporosis and are mired in autoimmune complications.

Review of the Effects of HDT on Bone Mass Density in Psychiatry

The psychiatric literature has a smaller database than the endocrine literature has. Four psychiatry publications showed no decrease in bone mass for patients treated with HDT. A 1997 cross-sectional study assessed 10 patients with rapid-cycling bipolar disorder treated with HDT and 10 controls. The average study time was six years. For the HDT group, TSH was suppressed below 0.4. The authors concluded that high-dose thyroid did not decrease bone mass density (Gyulai et al., 1997).

A cross-sectional study published in 2001 assessed the response of 26 affectively ill women (20 with bipolar disorder and six with major depression) equally divided between premenopausal and postmenopausal status, receiving HDT treatment. Premenopausal patients were treated for around three years, with a mean T4 dose of 281 mg/day and an average T4 blood level of 12.6 mcg/l. The postmenopausal women were treated for a mean of 6.8 years with an average dose of 356 mcg/day of T4, obtaining a mean T4 blood level of 14.3 mcg/l. There was no statistically significant change of bone mass density for either the pre- or postmenopausal women (Gyulai et al., 2001).

A prospective trial published in 2004 looked at the effects of high-dose T4 on 21 affectively ill patients; 13 of whom suffered with bipolar, four with major depression, and four with schizoaffective disorder. Bone mass density was first measured after an average treatment length of 16.4 months and again after an average of 33.6 months of therapy. The patients were receiving an average of a little over 400 mcg of T4. This high dose of T4 achieved high blood levels of circulating thyroid hormone. Measurements taken in both time periods were equivalent, showing significantly suppressed TSH and significantly high T3 and T4. There was no significant difference in bone mass density compared with that expected for the population. The authors reported that patients experienced considerable symptom improvement (Bauer et al., 2004).

The most recent psychiatric study, published in 2012, looked at twenty-two affectively ill patients compared with an age- and gender-matched group. The subjects were treated with high-dose T4 for an average of 5.8 years. HDT was not associated with any significant change in bone mass density. In this study, a fifty-nine-year-old male patient, who was diagnosed with osteopenia at baseline, had enough improvement in bone mass density to no longer be considered osteopenic. He received no formal treatment for osteopenia. The authors of the study believed that one of the main differences between hyperthyroid patients and psychiatric patients treated with HDT is that the psychiatric patients did not experience any thyrotoxic symptoms. The average blood levels were free T4 of 24.97 ng/l; total T3 of 1.74 ng/l, and a TSH of 0.06 mIU/L. For all but one of the 22 patients, the study was an extension of the 2001 Gyulai et al. study discussed above (Ricken et al., 2012b).

One psychiatric review paper looked at the safety of T3 use in patients suffering from major depression (Rosenthal et al., 2011). Unfortunately, it simply parroted the general warnings about the risks of HDT without actually examining any of the bipolar or the thyroid cancer literature.

HDT Used to Prevent the Return of Thyroid Cancer: Review of the Literature

A 2002 review by Quan and associates concluded that there was no risk of osteoporosis in men and premenopausal women. Quan concluded that the "findings for postmenopausal women remain unclear with two of the best controlled studies reporting opposing results." Quan cites a 1993 study done by Kung et al. as evidence that HDT may be a risk for osteoporosis in postmenopausal women. Quan overstates the results of the Kung et al. study. The conclusion stated in the Kung study is that HDT may cause a decrease of bone mass (Kung et al., 1993). The fact that women in China during this time period had extremely low dietary intake of calcium—on average, 500 mg/day—may have played a role in the bone loss.

The last review paper on this subject was published in 2006 by Heemstra et al.(Heemstra et al., 2006) Heemstra concluded that "our data suggest that postmenopausal women with subclinical hyperthyroidism (sic) are most at risk, whereas no increased risk was observed in men and premenopausal women." The "sic" was added because we saw earlier in the chapter that HDT does not fit the definition of hyperthyroidism. Heemstra's conclusion that postmenopausal women may be at risk for loss of bone mass contains critical errors that nullify the conclusion, and in fact, when reconsidered without the errors, the data point to the conclusion that HDT is not a risk factor for postmenopausal women.

Heemstra and associates based their conclusion that HDT is not a risk factor for men by reviewing eight studies. Two of the studies showed a decrease in bone mass density, and six showed no decrease in bone mass density.

For premenopausal women, 17 studies were examined, 12 showed no significant change in bone mass density, and five reported a decrease.

Postmenopausal women were included in 16 studies; the authors subdivided these into 14 cross-sectional studies and four longitudinal studies (two studies had both cross-sectional and longitudinal components). In the cross-sectional studies, only four showed a decrease in bone mass density, while 10 showed no decrease in bone mass density. In the longitudinal studies, two showed no change in bone mass density, and two, according to Heemstra, showed a decrease in bone mass density (Heemstra et al., 2006). Heemstra, while not explicitly stating so, appears to have placed the greatest emphasis on the two longitudinal studies that purported to show a decrease in bone mass density. However, Heemstra and associates erred in their examination of these studies. The first failed to meet Heemstra's stated criteria for inclusion. In the second study, Heemstra and associates plainly misquoted the results of a study, ignoring or failing to see that the study they were examining explicitly stated that the results do not show that postmenopausal women had significant bone loss. We will examine these two studies in detail.

The first longitudinal study cited by Heemstra, Kung and Yeung, studied 46 Chinese postmenopausal women. One of Heemstra's stated criteria for inclusion in the meta-analysis is that studies had to have a control group. In the Kung and Yeung study, there was no control group. In fact, Quan's earlier meta-analysis did not include Kung and Yeung's study for that very reason. In the study, the women were divided into three groups. The first group received supplementary calcium, calcitonin, and HDT; the second group received supplementary calcium and HDT; and the third group received a placebo and HDT.

Only women in the third group, with no supplementary calcium, showed a decrease in bone mass. Women with adequate calcium intake in the first two groups showed no decrease in bone mass. The addition of calcitonin made no difference. Effectively, the study only had one variable, low calcium versus adequate calcium intake. This makes it impossible to determine if HDT played a role in the loss of bone mass. Complicating this picture even more, the Chinese women in this study suffered from a lifetime of low dietary intake of calcium. Low calcium intake is a known risk factor for osteoporosis. In this study, the average dietary intake of calcium was just 508 mg a day, far below the recommended 1,200 mg/day (Kung and Yeung, 1996). Since low dietary calcium is a known risk factor for bone loss, it is more plausible that the low calcium intake was the cause of the decreased bone mass (Kung and Yeung, 1996). The Kung and Yeung study cannot be used to conclude that HDT causes bone loss.

The second longitudinal study that Heemstra cites to conclude that HDT is a risk for postmenopausal women was a 1998 study conducted by Jodar and associates (Jodar et al., 1998). Heemstra's review of Jodar's study is flawed in many ways, frankly contradicting Jodar's own conclusion. It is readily apparent that Heemstra fundamentally did not understand Jodar's study. The following errors were found:

1. In the longitudinal portion of the study, only one of five areas, the femoral neck, was purported to show a decrease in bone mass. The other four areas measured showed no significant bone loss.
2. Heemstra stated that in Jodar's longitudinal portion of the study, there were 39 postmenopausal women in the group. In

fact, the longitudinal portion only had a total of 27 women, and of these 27 women, only 13 were postmenopausal.
3. In the Jodar et al. study, the statistics that Heemstra cited were for both premenopausal and postmenopausal women lumped together. Jodar, in the longitudinal portion of the study, did not separately address postmenopausal women. Heemstra failed to recognize this. This alone negates Heemstra's conclusion.

Some may be tempted to reason that since there was no statistical difference between pre- and postmenopausal women, then the statistics for the whole group could be applied to postmenopausal portion. Since we don't have access to the separate data, there is no way to tell. With only 13 postmenopausal women and a fairly wide error margin, it is highly unlikely that there was a statistical difference in postmenopausal women in the longitudinal study. Numerically, postmenopausal women had less bone loss than premenopausal women. Normally, postmenopausal women have greater bone loss.

The most conspicuous mistake that Heemstra made was that his conclusion directly contradicts Jodar's conclusion with regard to the longitudinal study. Jodar specifically denied the significance of the longitudinal portion of the study findings regarding the femoral neck, stating, "Nevertheless, the minor changes in femoral neck bone mass density in our study in the face of the 1–2% in vivo coefficient of variation of DXA measures make this reduction unlikely to be meaningful" (Jodar et al., 1998).

On close inspection of the Heemstra et al. review paper, we see that there are no credible long-term studies showing that postmenopausal women are at risk for bone loss with HDT. This leaves us with two longitudinal studies showing no bone loss, 10 cross-sectional studies showing no bone loss, and four cross-sectional studies showing bone loss. The preponderance of evidence, the same method used by Heemstra in the rest of the review, justifies the conclusion that HDT does not significantly change bone mass for postmenopausal women.

It is interesting that as we look at the studies reviewed by Heemstra, there is a trend in the more modern studies not to show a decrease in bone mass density. Likely, the more modern studies were more rigorous and/or the methodology of measuring bone mass density had a smaller margin of error.

Only three endocrine studies have been published since the Heemstra review. A cross-sectional study published in 2008 of 66 patients, consisting of 11 men, 22 premenopausal women, and 33 postmenopausal women being treated with HDT to suppress the reoccurrence of thyroid cancer. This study reported that HDT did not result in significant bone mass density decreases in men, premenopausal women, or postmenopausal women. The average treatment length was 15 months (Eftekhari et al., 2008).

The Sugitani and Fujimoto study is the most recent study looking at the effects of HDT on bone mass. This was a randomized, prospective controlled trial conducted in Japan of women with thyroid cancer. The study compared 144 patients on T4 HDT, and 127 control patients on nonsuppressive T4 doses. The average TSH was 0.070 u/ml for women on HDT. Bone mass was measured only in one site, at baseline, at one, three, and five years after thyroid surgery. When women of all ages were considered, there was no decrease in bone mass density in any of the time periods compared with controls. Numerically, the mean T scores for the HDT group dropped less than those of the control group at one year. However, the authors expressed concerns about the decrease of bone mass density at the one-year mark in women over 50 taking HDT. They did not report any such concerns at the three- and five-year measurements (Sugitani and Fujimoto, 2011). Sugitani and Fujimoto did a number of curious things that make it problematic to give credence to the authors' concern about potential bone loss in women > 50:

1. Their findings in women >50 at one year appear to be an ad hoc calculation (based on the fact that the authors did not discuss it in their methods section or report separate demographics). The authors failed to report separate baseline characteristics (BMI, age, bone mass density, and T scores) for women over 50. Since Sugitani and Fujimoto used a separate analysis of women over 50, they should have provided separate demographics to know if the treatment group and the control group of women >50 were matched. Without baseline characteristics, it is impossible to know if the separate analysis was valid. This alone is sufficient to

question the validity of the concern of bone loss in women >50.
2. The authors did not directly compare T scores between groups but choose to compare the change from baseline to the one-year time period. In other words, they subtracted the one-year T score from the baseline T score within the treatment group and within the control group. (The fact that they did this only once in the entire paper also points to an ad hoc analysis.) They then compared scores. This artificially inflates the differences. This is statistical manipulation at its worst. If the changes were significant, a direct comparison between the treatment group T scores and the control group T scores, as the authors did for every other comparison, would have been valid.
3. The study did not control for thyrotoxic symptoms, vitamin D intake, physical exercise, or smoking. The two most important pieces of information they left out were the subjects' actual menopausal status and the number of years that the women were postmenopausal. Also important would have been the average dietary calcium intake. Japanese have a much lower calcium intake, on average, than do people eating Western diets. The authors did not use the potentially more useful z scores, which are the standard of research. This would particularly be important in Japan (z scores are based on countries or cultures) due to the low dietary calcium intake. This is also important because postmenopausal women have an increased rate of bone mass loss just prior to and immediately following menopause.
4. This study only measured one site. Single-site studies are considered less reliable. In studies that measure multiple sites, it is not unusual for one site to show a decrease while other sites show improvement or no change. Another concern is that 6% (n=10) of the treatment group dropped out of the study in the first year due to thyrotoxicity. This potentially indicates that the authors were rigid in their approach to the dosing of T4.

Curiously, the authors were mute on the fate of women over 50 at the three- and five-year measurements. Since they failed to report significant bone losses, we can only assume that the there was no significant bone loss and that their findings about women > 50 having bone loss at the one-year mark were either spurious, random, or specious, based on their artificial inflating of the differences. Alternatively, it implies that if there was a real difference at the one-year mark, then women > 50 had made up any bone loss by time they reached the third year. If HDT truly causes a decrease in bone mass density in women over 50, the three and five-year measurements would be much more revealing than the one-year measurements were. The fact that there was no significant bone loss for women over 50 at three and five years reinforces the conclusion that HDT is not a risk factor for bone loss for postmenopausal women. The fact that there was no significant bone loss for all women on HDT at five years reinforces the conclusion that HDT is not a risk factor for bone loss.

Here is another important point that was not considered in the study but lends strength to the conclusion that HDT is not a risk factor for postmenopausal women. The average age of menopause in Japan is 50.2 +/- 3.24 years (Kono et al., 1990). The average age of the women in the Sugitani and Fujimoto study at the beginning was 51.2 +/- 13.8 years. This would indicate that by the end of the five-year study a substantial majority of women would have been postmenopausal. Yet for all women, there was no statistical difference in bone mass density between treatment and control groups at the five-year measurement. Numerically, at the five-year measurement, the average T score dropped less for women treated with HDT than for women treated with just replacement doses of T4.

In sum, a multitude of problems with how Sugitani and Fujimoto evaluated and reported bone loss for women over the age of fifty on HDT renders any conclusions about women over 50 on HDT as scientifically invalid. The results of the three-year and five-year measurements points to the conclusion that HDT is not a risk factor for osteoporosis for women of any age. At the end of the five-year period, the majority of women were postmenopausal, yet they did not show significant bone loss when compared with controls. Instead of raising concerns about postmenopausal women, a close examination of the Sugitani and Fujimoto study lends support to the conclusion that HDT is not a risk factor for bone loss in postmenopausal women.

Bone-Turnover Markers

Bone-turnover markers, signifying remodeling of bones, are consistently cited as evidence that high levels of circulating hormone cause osteoporosis. Here is a study that shows HDT can cause elevated bone-turnover markers yet does not decrease bone mass. Further, the study shows that hyperthyroid women continue to lose bone mass and have increased bone markers even three years after their thyroid levels were normalized. Balaya and associates' study is the only study that directly and prospectively compared the effects of hyperthyroidism and HDT on bone mass and bone markers. The authors compared four groups of postmenopausal women: a group of patients treated with HDT for thyroid cancer, a normal control group (without any thyroid disturbances or cancer), a group of patients with Graves' hyperthyroidism, and a group with hyperthyroidism due to toxic multinodular goiter.

Both groups of patients suffering from hyperthyroidism had received antithyroid treatments before the start of the study that resulted in normal TSH, T3, and T4 levels for six months prior to the start of the study. Bone mass densities were evaluated at the beginning of the study and again after an average of three years of treatment. The group that suffered from thyroid cancer was treated with T4 HDT for at least three years, some longer. It is important to note that the thyroid cancer group was the only group to have high circulating thyroid levels during the study. The fourth group was a control group of thyroid-disease-free women. Both groups that had previously been hyperthyroid and the HDT treatment group had elevated bone-turnover markers, indicating an increase in osteoblast activity and a decrease in osteoclast activity. The bone mass densities decreased significantly in both hyperthyroid groups (despite the fact that they had normal TSH, T3, and T4 for the whole evaluation period and for six months prior to the study), yet the thyroid cancer group treated with HDT had no decrease in bone mass density despite having elevated bone markers (Belaya et al., 2007). This is rather a remarkable study with three important findings. They are that:

1. HDT does not cause bone loss;
2. bone-turnover markers are not necessarily connected with bone loss; and
3. hyperthyroidism continues to cause bone mass loss and elevated bone markers well after thyroid levels are normalized. This implies that whatever the process of bone loss connected with hyperthyroidism is:
   a. it is not connected with high thyroid levels; and
   b. it continues even after definitive treatment for hyperthyroidism has taken place.

The most likely cause for continued bone loss is the autoimmune process that continues even after thyroid ablation. See chapter 4 for further discussion.

What about Animal Studies Showing That HDT Causes a Decrease in Bone Mass?

Animal studies of HDT used doses of thyroid hormone far in excess of doses used by humans. For example, a study of female water eels were given the human equivalent of over 400,000 mcg of either T3 or T4 a day (Sbaihi et al., 2007). In a study by Kung and Ng, rats received the human equivalent of 15,000 to 45,000 mcg of T4 a day (Kung and Ng, 1994). In another study, rats were treated with the human equivalent of 18,750 mcg of T4 a day (Kono et al., 1990). In a more "reasonably" dosed study, rats were given the human equivalent of up to 1,500 mcg of T4 a day (Talaeipour et al., 2014). All of these studies indicated bone loss. There are a number of problems with generalizing these studies to the issues discussed in this book. They include the following:

1. These are massive doses. Thyroid hormones do have similarities to other biologically active compounds. Normally, these are not an issue, but these massive doses may trigger nonthyroidal receptors, or some of the thyroid hormone may be metabolized in sufficient quantities to other hormones that may have ill effects.
2. All three of the rat studies gave T4 intraperitoneally, which is better absorbed than oral T4 because it bypasses to some

degree the first-pass effects. This would make the effective doses even higher.
3. How generalizable are studies of rats and eels to humans? Especially considering the massive doses. Also, it is hard to get water eels to do weight-bearing exercises.
4. At the risk of anthropomorphizing, these massive doses likely made the rats or eels "feel" ill in some significant way that could have had an effect on bone mass. In other words, sick animals do not make good study subjects.
5. In the face of extensive human data, animal models are irrelevant.

What Happens to Patients Who Develop Osteopenia or Osteoporosis during HDT Treatment?

The number of women who developed osteopenia or osteoporosis in the Depression and Bipolar Clinic while on HDT has been in line with the expected number of patients in the general population. Not all of the women who developed osteopenia or osteoporosis were receiving HDT. Clinically, the women who were treated with HDT and developed osteopenia or osteoporosis over the years all remained on or were forced to resume HDT. With appropriate treatment, their bone mass either stabilized or improved.

Conclusion: The evidence base for HDT indicates that it does not decrease bone mass. Therefore, it is not a risk factor for osteoporosis.

Chapter 7: The Myth That High-Dose Thyroid Is a Cardiac Risk Factor

Facts are stubborn, but statistics are more pliable.
–Mark Twain

In short: There are no credible studies showing that HDT increases cardiac morbidity or mortality, nor is there any credible research showing that HDT increases overall mortality.

This chapter reviews and expands on "An Examination of Myth: A Favorable Cardiovascular Risk-Benefit Analysis of High-Dose Thyroid for Affective Disorders" (Kelly et al., 2013). Only studies that assessed the risk of HDT were considered. The reasons for excluding studies of hyperthyroid patients are discussed in chapter 4.

It is remarkable that with the exception of two perspectives studies, none of the literature tracked the mortality of HDT. These reported fewer deaths in the HDT group compared with the non-HDT group. These studies are discussed below.

To put things in the proper perspective, the following should be kept in mind. When compared with the general population, hyperthyroidism causes a 20% premature death rate. (Fazio et al., 2004).

In reviewing the literature, only six studies have looked at the risk of cardiac problems and/or early mortality in patients using HDT. Four studies found no indication that HDT increased cardiovascular risks or premature death. Two studies purported to find risks from HDT, but on closer examination, they failed to show any risk.

Of the four studies that showed no risk, the first and largest study, performed in Finland, followed 2,479 patients for an average of 16 years of treatment with HDT for thyroid cancer for a total of 39,664 patient years. There was no significant difference in the cardiovascular morbidity and mortality between the thyroid cancer group and the general public (Akslen et al., 1991).

A second study of HDT-treated patients was a multi-institute registry study with a median of three-year follow-up (range 0–14).

This study divided patients who had proven adherence to HDT therapy, n=1,548, demonstrated by repeated low TSH levels and patients who did not adhere to HDT treatment protocols n=1,388. This equaled 4,644 patient-years of HDT-treated patients. HDT treatment was shown to be beneficial to overall survival and to disease-specific survival for patients with stage II, III, and IV thyroid cancer. There was no difference in the overall survival of stage I thyroid cancer patients treated with HDT (n=681) compared with non-HDT-treated Stage I thyroid cancer control patients (n=611). Discounting the patients who died of a reoccurrence of the cancer, there were less than half as many deaths in the HDT group (1.9%) than in the non-HDT group (5.2%). This was a trend and did not reach statistical significance (Jonklaas et al., 2006).

The third study was of 504 Dutch patients followed for median of nine years, for an estimated 4,536 patient years of patients treated with HDT. It found no significant difference cardiovascular deaths compared with the general population. Nor was there any difference from all causes of death in individuals treated for thyroid cancer compared to the general population who did not have thyroid cancer reoccur (Links et al., 2005).

The fourth study, done by Sugitani and Fujimoto and discussed in the osteoporosis chapter, also evaluated cardiovascular mortality and overall mortality. The study followed 225 patients for five years. Roughly half of the patients were treated with HDT to prevent the return of thyroid cancer, and a control group of patients with thyroid cancer was treated only with replacement levels of thyroid hormone. This equals 600 patient years in the HDT group. There were no reported deaths from cardiovascular causes in either group. Three patients in the HDT group were dropped from the study due to unspecified cardiovascular disease. One patient from both groups died due to a reoccurrence of thyroid cancer. Excluding patients who died due thyroid cancer relapse, fewer of the HDT-treated group died (0.8%), while 3.8% of the control group died. No statistical evaluation was done on these figures (Sugitani and Fujimoto, 2011).

Only one study of 524 Dutch patients being treated for thyroid cancer described the possibility of increased cardiovascular deaths associated with HDT. The study's authors admit that bias introduced by their methods of comparison renders comparisons between the treatment group and the control invalid. The mean age at baseline was 49. The control group was the general public. This study has a number of major flaws that negate its scientific validity. Some of the flaws were acknowledged by the authors, and some were not. TSH levels were monitored, and the median follow-up time was 8.5 years. The authors reported a rate of 4.2% (n=22) cardiovascular related deaths with a calculated hazard ratio (HR) [sic] of 3.15 for cardiovascular death and 4.40 for all-cause mortality. The all-cause mortality included recurrence of thyroid cancer (Hesselink et al., 2013).

    The "sic" was included because the study incorrectly applied the use of HR. HR can only be used in comparing two similar groups. In order to calculate HR, the control group should have been thyroid cancer patients treated with replacement levels of thyroid hormone and tracked the same as the treatment group. Instead, in this study the "control group" was the general public. Much greater efforts were made to find the cause of death for the thyroid cancer patients, including a review of public records, hospital records, medical records, autopsy reports, and information from general practitioners. The comparison of general population deaths used only information available from public records. In this type of comparison, the actual difference between illnesses that are found incidentally and those that are specifically looked for can be profound. An example of this is obstructive sleep apnea (OSA). The estimate of the prevalence of OSA in those suffering from a bipolar disorder was 3.3%, based on information from a large Veterans Administration database. When patients were actively screened, the point prevalence of OSA was found to be at least 21% and perhaps as high as 47% (Kelly et al., 2013). The estimation of 47% was found also in one other study of OSA (Leboyer et al., 2012).

    The study's authors admit this method of comparison introduces a bias that makes comparisons invalid. Curiously, even though a comparison is not valid, they nonetheless make the comparison and then compound their error by calculating HRs. Further, a large number of patients were lost to follow-up; the death of even a few more patients from either the treatment or control groups could have altered the outcome if these individuals had been included in the final analysis. Interestingly, none of the patients with a known history of diabetes or heart disease in the HDT group died.

This is counterintuitive to the notion that HDT increases the risks of cardiovascular mortality. Important information needed to evaluate the deaths associated with HDT is missing, such as the ages of the patients or disease state. While the authors reported the number of patients who died from thyroid cancer recurrence, they did not report whether the patients who experienced cardiac death did so during a thyroid cancer recurrence. It is not unreasonable to suspect that patients weakened by thyroid cancer recurrence and associated treatments may be more vulnerable to cardiovascular-related deaths (Hesselink et al., 2013). Most importantly, given the four studies discussed above, when the control group and the treatment group were directly comparable, there was no indication that HDT causes increased cardiovascular mortality or increases mortality at all.

Only one paper, by Abonowara and associates (Abonowara et al., 2012), discussed whether the long-term use of HDT to prevent recurrence of thyroid cancer increased the risk of atrial fibrillation (AF). This study is deeply flawed. The study included 136 subjects who were followed for an average of 11 years. No deaths were reported for a total of 1,496 patient years. The mean TSH level was 0.17 mIU/L. A total of 14 patients were found to have AF—two with long-standing, persistent AF and 12 with paroxysmal AF. The authors compare these results with the rate of AF found in a population study done by Go(Go et al., 2001). The authors concluded that "TSH suppression in thyroid cancer is associated with a high prevalence of AF ($p < 0.0001$)." However, careful examination of this paper reveals numerous major flaws. These flaws not only negate the authors' conclusion, but if corrected, they actually contradict the authors' conclusion. The authors included in the study a patient with preexisting AF before HDT was started. This patient should have been excluded. The most egregious flaw was that the authors used a definition of AF that significantly differed from the definition used in the comparison paper. The comparison study by Go et al. excluded paroxysmal AF when reporting results (Go et al., 2001). Abonowara et al. include in their final count 12 patients with paroxysmal AF. If the Go et al. definitions were used, the 12 patients with paroxysmal AF should have been excluded. This would leave only two patients with AF. If the one case of persistent AF that was present before HDT treatment was excluded and the paroxysmal AF cases were excluded, the incidence of AF for patients treated for HDT was only 0.74% (n=1). The prevalence of AF in the comparison study of by Go et al. was 0.95%.

HDT possibly may have positive cardiac effects. Thyroid hormones are proangiogenic and stimulate arteriolar growth in normal hearts as well as in post myocardial infarction hearts (Biondi, 2012). Experimental and clinical evidence is showing a beneficial effect of the thyroid hormones on limiting cardiac ischemic injury, preventing post infarction cardiac remodeling, reversing post infarction cardiac remodeling, and improving cardiac hemodynamics (Pantos et al., 2010).

Cardiovascular Risks Found in the Psychiatric Literature

No studies that directly examined the risks of HDT in psychiatric patients could be found. In a 2001 review of HDT, Michael Bauer and Peter C. Whybrow stated, "However, there is no evidence from preliminary follow-up studies that the cardiovascular system is clinically impaired during supraphysiological T4 treatment in patients with affective disorders" (Bauer and Whybrow, 2001).

Case Reports of Atrial Fibrillation with HDT Treatment

There is one psychiatric paper that reported a small case series of AF associated with HDT (Kelly, 2015). These were patients at the Depression & Bipolar Clinic of Colorado. There well over 800 patients have been treated with long term HDT. Since the paper was published there has been one additional case of AF.

Six patients that I treated with HDT have developed AF. All of the patients who developed AF were being treated with T3 and diagnosed with bipolar II or bipolar not otherwise specified (NOS). In one case, HDT was continued, and the AF continued. In the five cases where the HDT was stopped or the dose greatly reduced, AF spontaneously remitted in less than three weeks. In all four cases where HDT was discontinued or the dose was greatly reduced, severe depression reemerged. In the three cases where HDT was resumed, the patients once again showed significant improvement.

The first case was a 50year-old female who had a prior history of AF; she had been treated with T3 for 10 project that months at a dose of 50 mcg. After stopping T3, she relapsed into a severe depression, with GAF scores ranging from 30 to 40. After multiple failures with other treatment augmentations, she, in consultation with her cardiologist and without consulting me, resumed HDT. At that time, I would have opposed a retrial of T3. With the HDT restored she became euthymic. Over the subsequent 2 years, her T3 dose was adjusted upward to almost double the dose that she had originally developed AF without a reoccurrence of AF.

The second case was a 35 yo male who developed AF after three months of treatment of T3 at 75 mcg. The patient's AF started after a day of heavy drinking (amount unknown), a large ingestion of methylphenidate (dose and source unknown), caffeine, dehydration, and extensive sun exposure—all while attending a baseball doubleheader. The AF remitted after the T3, alcohol, and methylphenidate were stopped. His bipolar depression returned, and he was soon lost to follow-up.

The third case was an 86 yo female who developed AF after 10 months of T3 treatment at 50 mcg per day. After consultation with her primary care physician and her family, the patient elected to stay on HDT because of the previous severity of her depression (GAF scores in the 30s). The patient, her family, her primary care physician, and I were convinced that if the HDT were stopped, at best her quality of life would be extremely poor, and at worse her depression would lead to death. She was prophylactically treated with anticlotting agents, and she has remained healthy with no complications associated with AF for nine years.

The fourth patient was a 55 yo female who developed AF after eight years of treatment with a final T3 dose of 167.5 mcg daily. After stopping T3, she relapsed into a severe depression that two further trials of other treatment agents failed to resolve. With the return of her severe depression, she developed suicidal ideation, gained 40lb, restarted cigarettes, and was demoted at work, a demotion that she directly attributed to the depression. She restarted HDT. After 10 months, the AF has not returned, and her depression improved but not to the degree that she enjoyed prior to stopping T3.

The fifth case of was a 62 yo male treated for 8.5 years with T3 at a daily dose of 87.5 mcg who developed AF during a hospitalization for pneumonia. He did not have the AF when he entered the hospital. Pneumonia is a known risk factor for AF (Soto-Gomez et al., 2013). The AF spontaneously remitted after T3 was stopped, and his pneumonia resolved. Severe depressive symptoms started to return after he was released from the hospital, and HDT treatment was restarted. There has been no return of AF in three years. The T3 dose has increased to 100 mcg.

The sixth patient was a 68 yo male who developed AF after seven years of T3 at a dose of 175 mcg. The T3 was stopped, and the AF remitted. His depression returned, and T3 was restarted and raised to a dose of 125 mcg. The previous benefits returned, and his depression remitted. Six months later, his AF returned. Despite multiple admonitions to minimize caffeine, he had restarted five cups or more a day of coffee. Instead of changing the T3 dose the patient was asked to stop all caffeine use. One week later, despite continuing one cup of coffee a day his AF was gone and not returned on close follow-up.

Was the HDT the Etiology of the AF?

It is difficult to draw firm conclusions from the six case reports. Whether or not HDT is used, there will be a certain percentage of patients who spontaneously develop AF as happens in the general population. The lifetime risk for developing AF is around 25%, according to the Framingham Heart Study (Hubert et al., 1983) and the point prevalence is 0.95% (Go et al., 2001). In five of six cases, there were known risk factors for AF, including advanced age (Heeringa et al., 2006), drug/alcohol abuse (Schelleman et al., 2012), pneumonia (Soto-Gomez et al., 2013), large caffeine intake, and a history of AF. The spontaneous remission of AF in all five of the patients who stopped T3 would indicate a causal relationship. However, this issue is clouded because of the four cases in which HDT was restarted, only one patient experienced a return of AF. In the one in whom AF did reoccur, greatly decreasing caffeine intake resulted in the remission of the AF. In the other three cases where depression returned and patients were forced to restart HDT, AF did not reemerge even in the face of higher doses of T3 than used prior to the development of AF. These cases highlight the complex nature of AF and the possibility that multiple risk factors were involved. Caffeine potentiates the heart rate effects of HDT (or HDT potentiates the heart rate effects of caffeine). Caffeine frequently needs to be stopped to keep the resting heart rate below 100 when higher doses of HDT are needed. Caffeine should be considered a risk factor in patients taking HDT, and its intake should be monitored.

Even if HDT is potentially a small risk factor for AF, the risk can be minimized by monitoring patients. This can easily be accomplished with a pulse oximeter with a wave form that facilitates monitoring for tachycardia and for an irregularly irregular heart rhythm, the hallmark of AF. In hyperthyroid subjects, the risks of developing more serious arrhythmias (e.g., atrial flutter, ventricular tachycardia, and paroxysmal supraventricular tachycardia) are uncommon (Fadel et al., 2000). In hyperthyroidism, AF spontaneously remits after treatment of the hyperthyroidism in the vast majority of cases, with the exception of the elderly, where it remits most of the time (Biondi and Kahaly, 2010; Fazio et al., 2004). The observations of no increase in the sudden cardiac death rate and, more importantly, no increase of all-cause mortality in HDT in the four studies discussed above suggest that the risk of ventricular fibrillation is minimal or absent.

These studies of HDT indicating no increase in mortality stand in stark contrast to the studies of hyperthyroidism that show a 20% premature death rate. The only studies that purported that long-term HDT may be associated with cardiac risk are deeply flawed.

No studies have directly assessed the cardiovascular risks of HDT in psychiatry patients.

How Serious Is Atrial Fibrillation?

If there is a risk of AF from HDT, then there are two questions that arise. The first is how serious is AF. In younger, healthy patients, it is not necessarily serious. There is some debate whether younger, healthy patients who develop AF even need to be treated with prophylactic blood thinners. The danger of AF increases in the presence of other cardiac risk factors. The second question that arises is how serious is it in psychiatric patients. Experience shows that when AF arises, simply by discontinuing HDT, decreasing the dose of HDT, and/or minimizing caffeine use, AF will remit and not return even when rechallenged with HDT when risk factors are controlled. In all six cases discussed above the riskbenefit analysis favored either staying on HDT or returning to HDT when other suspected etiologies have been controlled. Ongoing monitoring for tachycardia and/or serial EKGs can minimize the risk of AF. (See the section on monitoring recommendations.) Monitoring using a single-lead EKG is feasible in a psychiatrist's office and billable to insurance. It can be done with an iPhone and a Bluetooth device. The software can "read" the EKG. Questionable EKGs can be sent out for further analysis. Even without the software, it is fairly easy to recognize normal sinus rhythm or AF.

In the final analysis, the development of AF should trigger an analysis of other contributing factors, a risk-benefit analysis of stopping vs. continuing HDT, and, if need be, a taper of T3, monitoring for remission of the AF and monitoring for relapse mood difficulties. The taper can avoid the potential cardiac complications from abruptly discontinuing HDT and minimize the risk for precipitating a severe relapse. Patients who develop AF must be evaluated on an individual basis. Experience suggests that the HDT dose can be decreased or stopped long enough for the AF to stop and later restarted, if needed. The risk-benefit analysis may well indicate continuing on HDT even if the AF can't be reversed. HDT should be continued with seriously affectively ill individuals who have received substantial benefit from HDT—particularly patients who have exhausted alternative treatments or for whom the alternative treatments would carry a greater risk than AF does (e.g., using Seroquel in a brittle diabetic).

Summary: Four of the six studies discussed above (five, if you include the corrected paper on AF) do not indicate any increased risk to the heart or premature death. This is based on an estimated 50,940 patient years of HDT with no increase in mortality. (One study reported medium years, and this number was substituted for the mean to arrive at the estimate.)

The only studies that purported that long-term HDT may be associated with cardiac risk are deeply flawed.

There are reasons to believe that if any risks do exist, these risks would be less for affective illness than for thyroid cancer patients (see chapter 13). Further, HDT may actually decrease the morbidity or mortality of the medical problems of the bipolar disorder. While the research indicates that HDT seems to be at least as safe as or safer than many of our psychiatric medications, specific medical problems and advanced age may preclude the use of HDT—or for that matter, may exclude other psychiatric medications. A careful assessment of the risks vs. benefits of any medical treatment is always required. The high morbidity and mortality associated with less-than-fully controlled bipolar disorders is not to be ignored or discounted. Likewise, the considerable risk from alternative medicines that we may use, as we will see in the next chapter, cannot be ignored or discounted.

Chapter 8: The Risks of Other Psychiatric Medications and the Undertreatment of Bipolar Disorders

> Risk is like fire: If controlled it will help you; if uncontrolled it will rise up and destroy you.
> –Theodore Roosevelt

Summary: HDT is as safe as or safer than most psychiatric medications. A risk vs. risk analysis of HDT vs. other potential bipolar medications is highly favorable toward HDT.

All treatments come with risks. The scope of this chapter is to assist in the development of a risk-benefit analysis of HDT by surveying the risks of other psychiatric medications used to treat the bipolar disorders, the risks of no treatment, and the risk of undertreatment. While HDT should not be considered risk-free, the risks of HDT by in large compare very favorably to the risks of other medications used to treat the bipolar disorders. The potential severe side effects, morbidity, and mortality of bipolar medications will be examined. This chapter should not be considered an exhaustive review of the risk of psychiatric medications.

Risks vs. Benefits: Risks of Psychiatric Medications

Untreated or undertreated bipolar disorders carry considerable risks that are far greater than treatment. The risks are not just limited to the patient alone. Untreated patients with a bipolar disorder are a drain on their families and society in general. Untreated patients with a bipolar disorder can pose a considerable risk of danger to others. Partially controlling the symptoms of a bipolar disorder still carries a substantial risk, primarily the through the risk of a relapse and the not insignificant drain over time of residual symptoms. This chapter is divided into six sections. The first section will briefly discuss the risks of failing to achieve full remission. The second section discusses the risks of osteoporosis from psychiatric medications, and the third section will discuss the morbidity and mortality of psychiatric medications. The fourth section discusses weight gain, and the fifth discusses the risks associated with sedating medications. The sixth and last section covers the risks associated with Li, valproic acid, carbamazepine, and lamotrigine. This chapter does not address the myriad of nagging side effects that have negative impacts on our patients' lives.

Failure to Treat Bipolar Disorder

Failure to adequately treat bipolar disorders carries significant risks that far outweigh the risks of medications. Bipolar disorders carry a high risk of suicide. The absolute risk of suicide among patients with a diagnosis of BD is around 8% for men and 5% for women. Over a median of 18 years' follow-up, the suicide risk for people with BD compared with that in the general population has been reported to be 10–30 fold greater. Rates of suicide attempts are far higher, with an estimated annual risk of 0.9% per year, and a 50% lifetime risk of an attempt. As we know, some suicide attempts are minimal and have no lasting impact on the patient's health. But a not insignificant number of suicide attempts leave patients with permanent disabilities. No information could be found in the literature to indicate how often this is the case. A recent meta-analysis of over 75,000 bipolar patients showed 1,149 suicide deaths (2%) (Schaffer et al., 2015). However, the patients studied were in active treatment or followed in research of some type. The rate of suicides is likely far higher than this. How many of our patients get discouraged, drop out of treatment, and then suicide? How many patients suicide before they are even seen in treatment? For that matter, how many psychiatric patients suicide with an unrecognized bipolar disorder?

On average, patients suffering a bipolar disorder die 10 to 20 years earlier than the general population. Surprisingly, suicide plays only a small role in the premature death rate (Osby et al., 2001). The medical morbidity and mortality of the bipolar disorders are considerable. It is estimated that 58% of individuals with a bipolar disorder have a comorbid medical conditions(Magalhaes et al., 2012). Many forms of heart disease, hypertension, angina, tachycardia, atherosclerosis, and myocardial infarction are more prevalent than in the general population. Individuals suffering from bipolar disorders experience the onset of cardiovascular disease an average of thirteen years early. Arthritis, gastritis, other diseases of the stomach, cirrhosis of the liver, and other forms of liver disease all more prevalent in people suffering a bipolar disorder (Frye et al., 2011). Given the more recent recognition that obstructive sleep apnea affects an estimated 47% of patients with a bipolar disorder, it is likely that there is a higher rate of comorbid medical problems associated with the bipolar disorders than previously suspected (Kelly et al., 2013; Leboyer et al., 2012). It is likely that people with bipolar II and the other spectrum bipolar illnesses suffer the same degree of medical problems and possibly worse. Bipolar depressions are associated with repeated episodes of decreased physical activity and nutritional abnormalities—both known risks for osteoporosis. Inactivity is considered the largest risk factor for osteoporosis. It is not uncommon for a bipolar II depressed patient to spend twelve to fourteen hours sleeping and a couple more hours on the couch. Tobacco and alcohol are known risk factors for osteoporosis, and both are more prevalent in patients suffering a bipolar disorder (Halbreich et al., 1995).

Obesity is a big problem for many patients. According to the Centers for Disease Control and Prevention (CDC), bipolar costs the United States $6.85 billion a year in direct expenses, disability payments, and lost productivity. The total cost to society is at least $56 billion dollars a year, adjusted for inflation (Hirschfeld et al., 2005). This is certainly an underestimation. It is difficult to estimate all of the costs. What is the cost to society of unrecognized bipolar disorder? What are the costs of irritability leading to violence? What are the costs of impulsivity and daredevil activities that result in destruction of property, injury, or death? While no research could be located regarding the risk of nonsuicide-related injuries or death to self or others associated with the bipolar disorders, there can't be any doubt that these are of considerable cost to society. Nor can we estimate the cost and the number of deaths or injuries caused by inattentive or quasisuicidal depressed patients. The toll on family and friends is incalculable. Irritability is a constant drain on families and those who interact with an individual with bipolar disorder. There are hidden medical costs: many bipolar patients have multiple physical complaints that just can never be pinned down, and they undergo repeated medical workups. The overactivity of hypomania can have lasting effects. Clinically, it is not unusual to find patients who have spent extended periods hypomanic, have all but ruined their bodies due to extreme exercise (e.g., running 10 miles or more a day, seven days a week for decades) leaving these patients all but crippled with degenerative arthritis and injuries. Overexercise or excessive exercise leaves patients vulnerable to injuries in general, particularly injuries associated with repetitive motion.

What is the percentage of unrecognized or untreated bipolar individuals in jails? One study utilizing only the Mood Disorder Questionnaire (MDQ) estimated unrecognized bipolar at 13% in a prison. There are certainly much higher percentages than this, as the MDQ is notoriously bad at recognizing bipolar II and bipolar NOS. Based on three years of experience at a local jail, clinical estimates predicted 30% of the inmates suffer from an unrecognized or untreated bipolar disorder. A full-time psychologist who had worked at the jail for over a decade estimated 50%. The vast majority were unrecognized bipolar II or NOS, whose chief symptom was not euphoria but irritability. Their behavior during hypomanic or mixed episodes directly led to repeated incarcerations. This exacerbates and accelerates the spiral down the socioeconomic ladder that often companies the bipolar disorders. Incarceration exacerbates alcohol and drug use that is already high due to the bipolar disorder.

Risk of Osteoporosis from Psychiatric Medications

Many of the commonly used treatments for the bipolar disorders pose a risk for osteoporosis. Carbamazepine and valproic acid are both associated with a significant risk for osteoporosis (O'Connell et al., 2010). Serotonin reuptake inhibitors carry a risk for osteoporosis (Bruyère and Reginster, 2015). On the other hand, tricyclic antidepressants appear to be protective (Diem et al., 2007). Despite the common wisdom that selective serotonin reuptake inhibitors (SSRI) are safer for the elderly, there are fewer fractures associated with tricyclics than with SSRIs (Diem et al., 2007).

Neuroleptic medications have been associated with a significant risk of osteoporosis (Vestergaard, 2008). This is particularly true for patients treated with long-term, prolactin-raising antipsychotic medications (Meaney et al., 2004). Certainly, antipsychotics that cause orthostatic hypotension, balance problems,

Parkinson's side effects, gait abnormalities, or sedation increase the risk of falling and fractures as well as other problems outlined below.

Lithium is sometimes cited as being a risk factor for osteoporosis, but other papers report lithium use as neutral or protective of bone mass (Vestergaard, 2008; Zamani et al., 2009). However, if you don't carefully monitor thyroid levels (or use HDT), lithium can and often does cause a lowering of thyroid levels and even frank hypothyroidism. Hypothyroidism is a significant risk factor for osteoporosis.

Morbidity and Mortality Risks of medications

In evaluating mortality risks psychiatric medications, a comparison to cigarette smoking helps put things in perspective. Adjusted hazard ratios for all-causes death in smokers compared with those who never smoked were 1.3 for smokers of less than 10 cigarettes per day and 1.8 for those who smoked more than 10 cigarettes a day (Jacobsen and Comas-Díaz, 1999). Unfortunately, risks are reported in a variety of ways, making comparisons problematic.

Risk Associated with Tricyclics, SSRIs, and MAOI Antidepressants

Aside from the risks that antidepressants present to patients with bipolar disorders, there are considerable other risks. SSRIs are not associated with coronary heart disease, but they are associated with increased stroke risk, hazard ratio (HR) 1.45 and an even higher risk for fatal strokes, HR 2.12. SSRIs carry an all-cause mortality HR of 1.32. The HR for sudden cardiac death in patients on SSRIs was 3.34. Other studies have reported that SSRIs may decrease coronary artery disease (Narayan and Stein, 2009). Monoamine oxidase inhibitors carry a multitude of risks due to food and drug interactions, some potentially lethal. Certainly, the weight gain associated with some monoamine oxidase inhibitors can cause health problems. Severe serotonin syndrome is most associated with monoamine oxidase inhibitors and carries a high mortality rate (Deyuan, 2009). Tricyclic antidepressant use is associated with increased risk of mortality from any cause, (HR 1.67). The risk of overdose with tricyclics is considerable. Before the widespread use of SSRIs, tricyclics were involved in 15% to 33% of fatal poisonings in the United Kingdom. Likewise, in the past in the United States, tricyclics accounted for 37% of all poison-related admissions to intensive care (Thanacoody and Thomas, 2003). Tricyclics have been associated with torsade de pointes and other arrhythmias (Vieweg and Wood, 2004).

Antipsychotics

A significant risk of cardiac death was found for antipsychotics in a retrospective study of 481,744 Tennessee Medicaid patients (1,282,896 patient years). With moderate antipsychotic doses, the sudden cardiac death rate was 2.39 times greater than in nonusers, even when smoking and other health risks associated with serious mental illness were controlled for. This rate was only slightly reduced when schizophrenia was excluded (Ray et al., 2001).

Another large retrospective study (24,589 patient years) also found that antipsychotic use was a significant risk for sudden cardiac death. The authors went out of their way to control for confounding factors. They excluded deaths from other causes and any deaths that occurred during hospitalization or within 30 days of discharge. The control group was comprised of other mentally ill individuals who were not taking antipsychotics. The authors corrected the results for medically confounding factors, including smoking; other cardiovascular factors; somatic diseases; use of proarrhythmic medications; behavioral risk factors; substance abuse; poor self-care; and other effects of mental illness. The incident rate ratios for sudden death for specific drugs were: haloperidol, 1.61; thioridazine, 3.19; typical antipsychotics, 1.99; atypicals, 2.26; clozapine, 3.67; olanzapine, 2.04; quetiapine, 1.88; and risperidone, 2.91. Again, these were only slightly decreased when schizophrenia was excluded. The incidence-rate ratios of atypical agents ranged from 1.59 to 2.86 for low to high doses. Patients previously treated with antipsychotics did not have a significant risk of sudden cardiac death (Ray et al., 2001).

There are reports of sudden death associated with neuroleptic use (Ray et al., 2001). In patients residing in nursing homes, neuroleptics are associated with a small increased risk of death, and the use of neuroleptics in nursing homes has all but stopped.

Many antipsychotics cause concentration problems accompanied by EEG slowing.

Although rare, neuroleptic malignant syndrome has a high mortality rate (De-yuan, 2009).

Clozapine users have a 1% risk of developing agranulocytosis during the first year of treatment (Package-Insert). Agranulocytosis is often fatal (Woolcott et al., 2009). The incidence of myocarditis with clozapine ranges from one in 500 to one in 10,000. Clozapine-related cardiomyopathy, while rare, carries a 38% mortality rate (Tanner and Culling, 2003). Clozapine has been linked, in the first year of use, with seizures in 5% of patients, according to the package insert.

Sedating Medications

Patients are not always aware that sedation is associated with many psychotropic medications, nor are they always fully aware of its presence. Sedating psychotropic medications are associated with an increased risk of motor vehicle accidents (MVAs). High-potency sleep medications (e.g., zolpidem, zopiclone, eszopiclone, and zaleplon) have an adjusted odds ratio (OR) for motor vehicle accidents of 2.1. The OR for benzodiazepines is 2.09. Lower doses of antipsychotics carry an adjusted OR of 1.31 for motor vehicle accidents. Surprisingly, the OR for higher doses of antipsychotics is lower, with an adjusted OR of 0.92 (Chang et al., 2013).

Another study looked at the risks of motor vehicle accidents (MVA) with various sedating medications. In the first four weeks of benzodiazepine use, the incidence-rate ratio for MVAs was 1.94. After the first four weeks, the incidence-rate ratio increased to 2.38. The incidence-rate ratio for MVAs for SSRIs is 1.16. For antihistamines, the incidence rate ratio was 1.21. For comparison, opioid use had a incidence rate ratio for MVAs of 1.70–2.06 (Gibson et al., 2009). It should be kept in mind that MVAs are the tip of the iceberg in our patients' lives. Patients, like the rest of us, climb up to roofs, climb ladders, walk on ice, wake up in the middle of the night stumbling about, trip over dogs, step on cats, get up on chairs to change lightbulbs, or any number of unwise activities where sedation has the potential to create a disaster. This brings up the issue of equilibrium and dizziness as risk factors. The risk of falling is not just confined to the elderly. Most of the sedating medications can cause balance problems.

Sedative/hypnotics increase the risks of falling by 47%; antipsychotics increase fall risk 59%, and antidepressants, including SSRIs, increase fall risk by 68% (Woolcott et al., 2009).

While no literature addressed this, clinically, over 40% of bipolar depressed patients have significant problems with sedation (HDT does not cause sedation). This is more than would be expected just based on the medications alone.

In other words, the "sedation" from depression magnifies or is at least additive to the sedation from medications and likely is more dangerous. This seems logical in patients who are already suffering from sleep deprivation, concentration problems, or fatigue caused by their bipolar depression. The same observation has been made regarding cognitive problems—that is, patients already suffering cognitive problems from their bipolar illness will have a greater cognitive worsening than nondepressed individuals on the same medications—again, increasing the risk of these medications.

Weight Gain

Many psychotropic medications increase weight. Weight gain is associated with significant mortality and morbidity, greatly increasing the risk of many health problems such as cardiovascular disease, diabetes, obstructive sleep apnea, or other of the numerous weight-related illnesses (Frye et al., 2011). When treating patients with a bipolar disorder, it is hard to avoid medications that cause weight gain. In the general male population younger than 50 yo with high body mass index (BMI) values had twice the risk of coronary heart disease compared with those with low BMIs. Similarly, the risk is 2.4 times higher among obese women of the same age. Higher BMI values were associated with higher risks for sudden death in all age groups. The incidence of congestive heart failure in subjects younger than 50 is 2.5–3 times higher for the heaviest subjects. Women less than 70 years old with high BMI values had a fourfold higher stroke rate compared with the leanest group (Hubert et al., 1983). In addition to cardiovascular risk, weight gain also increases the incidence and severity of sleep apnea. This is important, given that the risk for obstructive sleep apnea (OSA) is already high in subjects with bipolar disorders, with estimates of 47% (Kelly et al., 2013; Leboyer et al., 2012). Patients taking tricyclics gain 1.3 to 2.9 pounds a month with an average gain of 16 pounds. Patients often abruptly stop tricyclics because of weight gain (Berken et al., 1984). The abrupt cessations of antidepressants can cause many problems, ranging from mild withdrawal to suicide.

Lithium, Valproic Acid, Tegretol, and Lamotrigine

Lithium-treated patients frequently gain 5% or more of their baseline weight (Fagiolini et al., 2002). In addition to weight gain, lithium has a myriad of other potential problems. Death or permanent neurological sequelae can result from lithium poisoning.

The mortality due to lithium overdose ranges from 1% to 15% (Bailey and McGuigan, 2000; Boeker et al., 2011). In acute overdose, one study estimated that 10% of survivors suffer permanent neurological sequelae (Boeker et al., 2011). Chronic lithium poisoning is far more dangerous. It is not unusual in clinical practice to find patients who start taking nonsteroidal anti-inflammatory medications or diuretics despite repeated warnings not to do so. Chronic lithium poisoning carries a considerably higher risk of severe neurotoxicity than an acute lithium overdose, (OR 6.20). In fact 92.9% of severe lithium neurotoxicity is directly attributable to chronic lithium poisoning (Oakley et al., 2001). Chronic Li poisonings are usually iatrogenic, either caused by inappropriate lithium dosing or concurrent use of medications that raise lithium levels such as nonsteroidal anti-inflammatory drugs, angiotensin-converting enzyme inhibitors, or angiotensin-II receptor antagonists (Cheng and Chong, 2013). Thiazide diuretics, by inducing sodium depletion, can lead to a 25% reduction of lithium clearance in just a week of therapy (Yip and Yeung, 2007). Age plays an important role in the development of severe lithium neurotoxicity, with an adjusted OR of 6.2 for individuals over 51 (Oakley et al., 2001). Unfortunately, nonpsychiatric physicians are, for the most part, unaware that these medications can pose a high danger to lithium users.

Lithium is detrimental to thyroid gland functioning in up to 50% of patients. Lithium concentrates in the thyroid gland, where it retards iodine uptake and impairs iodotyrosine coupling and hormone secretion. Li interferes with the conversion of T4 to T3 in the brain and alters the structure of thyroglobulin. Any alterations of the hypothalamic-pituitary-thyroid axis, even minor changes, have the potential to exacerbate the course of bipolar disorders. Studies have shown that lithium induces frank hypothyroidism in about 10% of individuals (range 0–47%) and induces subclinical hypothyroidism in about 25% (range 5–35%). Li can adversely affect the hypothalamic-pituitary-thyroid axis in ways other than the reduction of thyroid levels (Chakrabarti, 2011). Any drop in thyroid hormone levels, even if the levels remain within normal limits, is associated with more affective episodes and greater severity of depression during the first year of lithium treatment (Frye et al., 1999). Worse thyroid dysfunction significantly increases the risk for the development of lithium neurotoxicity, adjusted OR 9.3 (Oakley et al., 2001).

The majority of patients on lithium have EEG changes, mainly slowing. Normal volunteers taking Li have the same EEG slowing. Cognitive side effects, weight gain, and lack of coordination often lead to noncompliance. Tremor affects up to 65% of patients treated with lithium. Long term Li use can cause a decrease in renal functioning. Lithium overdose, especially chronic lithium poisoning, can have significant and lasting impact on renal functioning. Diabetes insipidus, characterized by a lack of response of the kidneys to antidiuretic hormone, occurs in approximately 10% of patients treated with lithium (Thanacoody and Thomas, 2003). When Li is combined with HDT, the risk of a significant tremor is higher and does not necessarily indicate toxicity from either Li or HDT.

Severe problems with Depakote (valproic acid) while rare, are significant (e.g., thrombocytopenia, hepatic failure, and hyperammonemia can lead to death if they occur). Pancreatitis is a potentially life-threatening event and described by many patients as the most painful experience they have ever had. Valproic acid causes pancreatitis in 1.5% of patients and can elevate serum amylase levels in 19% of individuals. Pancreatitis related to valproic acid use will reoccur 70% of the time if rechallenged (Yazdani et al., 2002). Incidence of fatal hepatotoxicity from valproic acid ranges from one in 8,312 to one in 15,517. The younger the age, the greater the risk. Polypharmacy increases the risk (Bryant and Dreifuss, 1996). It is recommended that liver enzymes been checked every six months. However, the idiosyncratic nature of these problems makes it difficult to catch on routine screening. Hair loss with valproic acid is not uncommon and not well-tolerated by patients with long hair.

Stevens-Johnson Syndrome and Toxic Epidermal Necrolysis

Serious and sometimes fatal dermatologic reactions, Stevens-Johnson syndrome and toxic epidermal necrolysis, have been estimated to occur in one to ten patients per 10,000 for both carbamazepine and lamotrigine. This risk is greatly increased with rapid dose escalation. Stevens-Johnson syndrome and toxic epidermal necrolysis are also possibilities with valproic use, but they occur at a lower rate than with carbamazepine and lamotrigine (Mockenhaupt et al., 2005)

While no studies of the sedation risks of valproic acid and carbamazepine could be located, sedative effects are often a problem. Cognitive problems are common also. It would seem likely that the sedative effects pose some risk for MVAs and other injuries.

Nagging Side Effects

Risks may cause a patient not to try a medication, but side effects are the most common reason patients stop taking medications. While this chapter does not attempt to cover the myriad of nagging side effects that negatively affect the lives of our patients, they nonetheless must be considered when choosing a medication. The nagging side effects can and do lead to a decreased quality of life; noncompliance with treatment; or worse, dropping out of treatment all together. While no head-to-head comparison trials have been conducted, clinically, most patients don't experience many, if any side effects from HDT. When they do, the side effects generally are mild or are easily handled by decreasing the dose.

Conclusion

The potential side effects of HDT are few and affect far fewer patients than most of the other medications we routinely use to treat bipolar disorders. Just having a treatment that isn't associated with weight gain, sedation, Stevens-Johnson syndrome, TD, sudden death, suicide, lithium toxicity, and a myriad of nagging side effects is intriguing all by itself. HDT is certainly far safer than leaving bipolar disorders undertreated or even partially treated. Based on these factors alone, HDT should be seriously considered early in treatment.

In addition, HDT has some intriguing prospects. The hypothesis of how HDT works (chapter 12) raises some exciting possibilities of how HDT may have added health benefits that could decrease the morbidity and mortality of bipolar disorder above and beyond just stabilizing the bipolar disorders.

Chapter 9: Is HDT a Risk Factor for Mania?

I have spent my life going from mania to mania. Somehow it has all paid off.
—Ray Bradbury

The short answer: Is HDT a risk factor for hypomania or mania? No. There are a limited number of case reports of hyperthyroidism causing mania. These case reports are weak. There are no case reports of HDT causing hypomania or mania.

There is some concern that "hyperthyroidism" or thyrotoxicosis can cause mania in patients with bipolar disorder. Keep in mind that HDT can never cause hyperthyroidism, and the likelihood that HDT would cause thyrotoxicity is low. It may cause a thyrotoxic symptom or two, but one or two mild symptoms are not thyrotoxicity. When thyrotoxic symptoms are detected, the thyroid dose is generally decreased. HDT will usually lead to high blood levels of thyroid hormones, but as per officially accepted definitions, high circulating levels alone are insufficient to be considered hyperthyroid or thyrotoxic. This may seem like splitting hairs, but as discussed in chapters 3 and 4, it is an important distinction with a difference. Understanding that HDT is relatively safe and does not cause hyperthyroidism gives us the impetus to look at these case reports in a new light.

Does Hyperthyroidism or Thyrotoxicity Cause Mania?

Most textbooks recommend that hyperthyroidism must be ruled out before mania is officially diagnosed. Yet case reports for mania associated with hyperthyroidism or thyrotoxicosis are extremely rare. Only four actual case reports of mania could be located, and one case report of a hypomania. There are papers that claim more reports, but when the citations are examined, many of these "reports" were not actual cases or they referred to one of four mania cases discussed here. Note that all of the following case reports involve patients with hyperthyroidism or subclinical hyperthyroidism; none were being treated with thyroid hormone supplementation:

1. A 2001 case report described a 65 yo male who initially developed a depressive episode for 11 days then developed mania. Both T3 and T4 were mildly elevated, but TSH, by today's standard, was normal. His mania improved with lorazepam as the sole treatment, and his hyperthyroidism was treated with a thyroid-suppressive agent. No further bipolar symptoms returned for the nine months that he was observed. There were no reported signs and symptoms of thyrotoxicosis reported in this case (Nath and Sagar, 2001).
2. A 1979 letter to the editor reported that a 43 yo female who was grossly thyrotoxic and apparently manic was treated with propranolol and propylthiouracil. Her manic symptoms decreased as her thyroid levels decreased. There was no past history of psychiatric illness. She had no psychiatric follow-up (Villani and Weitzel, 1979).
3. A 1983 case report described a 46 yo female who had had asymptomatic hydrocephalus since birth and developed mania and concomitantly high thyroid levels. She was treated with haloperidol and recovered fully. Her thyroid levels spontaneously normalized. She was well for four years and had a hypomanic episode (without elevation of thyroid levels) that remitted with haloperidol. She was well for another year and developed a frank mania with an elevated T4 but a normal T3. She recovered when treated with haloperidol. Her thyroid levels normalized (Corn and Checkley, 1983).
4. A 1991 case report described a 29 yo woman who developed mania with Graves' hyperthyroidism. In an ABAB experiment, she was treated with propranolol for five days, and her manic symptoms significantly decreased. When propranolol was withdrawn, her symptoms worsened. When propranolol was again restarted, her mania went into remission. Her hyperthyroidism was definitively treated, and she did not have a reoccurrence of mania (Lee et al., 1991).

These case reports, except for the last one, are rather sketchy on details—for example, case 2 had no follow-up; and in case 3, the patient sometimes had symptoms without elevated thyroid levels. To my knowledge, there has only been one reported case of hypomania secondary to hyperthyroidism. It was reported that the patient had no prior psychiatric history. Given the difficulty of correctly identifying bipolar II prior episodes, it may be difficult to identify prior episodes. The report did not have any long-term follow-up.

There are no case reports of HDT causing mania or hypomania in the thyroid cancer literature. If HDT were to cause mania or hypomania, it would be most likely to occur when HDT is used to treat bipolar disorder. Yet there are no case reports in the bipolar treatment literature. There are no case reports of when HDT was used to treat rapid cycling.

There are three issues. First, can patients with preexisting bipolar disorder develop mania when they become hyperthyroid? Second, can hyperthyroid patients develop mania that is unrelated to bipolar disorder? Third and most important, can HDT cause mania in bipolar patients?

Most of the case reports follow patients for a short time, making it more difficult to form a complete picture. Some reported cases didn't involve thyrotoxicity, just elevated thyroid levels. It is not impossible for bipolar disorder to have a late onset. Some cases involved other factors (e.g., hydrocephalus). Bipolar disorder and hyperthyroidism are not uncommon illnesses, so at least some incidental co-occurrence should be expected.

Given that levels are routinely drawn on psychiatric admission and when starting patient care with a psychiatrist and given the interest in this subject, it seems likely that if there is a causal link, there would be more case reports. There are too few reports to draw any definitive conclusions on any of these issues. While it is by no means conclusive, we can infer from the paucity of reports that neither hyperthyroidism nor HDT is a risk factor for developing hypomania or mania.

Chapter 10: The Use of HDT During Pregnancy and Breastfeeding

In short: HDT is at least relatively safe during pregnancy. Some experts, though not all, believe that T3 HDT without some added T4 may present a risk to developing fetuses. These risks are easily negated by using 150 mcg of T4 if using T3. Thyroid hormone may be released in sufficient quantities in lactation. The risk, if present, can be controlled for.

The FDA places liothyronine in pregnancy category A. This is the "safest" FDA category. Safest is in quotation marks because the FDA stopped using risk letter categories in 2015, as they were misleading for some medications (https://www.drugs.com/pregnancy-categories.html). Thyroid hormone is minimally transferred to the fetus thanks to the liver-like actions of the placenta. No studies have shown any adverse effects to the fetus.

Hyperthyroidism is dangerous to fetuses, but the danger is not because of high circulating levels of thyroid hormone. The placenta, once it starts to function at around 20 weeks of gestation, effectively protects the fetus from high thyroid levels. The same thyroid-receptor antibodies that cause hyperthyroidism in mothers readily pass through the placenta and cause hyperthyroidism in the developing fetuses. There is a positive association between the presence of thyroid antibodies (with or without hyperthyroidism) and pregnancy loss. For pregnant patients in need of HDT to protect from a reoccurrence of thyroid cancer, both the Endocrine Society and the American Thyroid Association recommend the use of HDT (De Groot et al., 2012).

It is interesting to note that T3 up to 50 mcg is sometimes used to treat euthyroid women who are experiencing difficulty conceiving or have had repeated miscarriages.

T3 vs. T4 in Pregnancy

Certain perinatal endocrinologists hold that the fetal brain can only absorb T4 before the fetus's own thyroid gland starts to function. The evidence backing this claim is weak but sufficient enough that using 150 mcg along with T3 is the best course.

Neonatologists don't agree with the above. They believe that fetuses are able to absorb T3 and are not concerned about high-dose T3. Clinically, there have been no negative consequences seen with the three patients who delivered normal children while taking high doses of T3 throughout pregnancy and breastfeeding. Their pregnancies and deliveries were normal. The children have reached normal developmental milestones. However, it is best to proceed with caution. It appears safest to discuss the need for some T4 during pregnancy, and 150 mcg of T4 can be substituted for 37.5 mcg of T3. Many women elect to be treated with T3 only.

Before Pregnancy

Keeping in mind the risks to fetuses, each woman of childbearing age should have a risk-benefit analysis performed at least once a year for all of medications currently in use. Since birth control methods fail at varying rates, if possible, these women should use medications considered safe for pregnancy. Having said that, it is often impossible to avoid medications that pose at least some teratogenic risk.

The Risk of Bipolar Disorder and Pregnancy

The largest risk during pregnancy often is the bipolar illness itself. Some women, because of the seriousness of their illness, must stay on medications. Bipolar depression is associated with a high rate of miscarriage, preterm labor, and small-for-gestational-age infants. Women with an untreated bipolar disorder are more likely to smoke, more likely to abuse substances, less likely to eat right, less likely to receive prenatal care during pregnancy, and more likely to be physically abused and not care for themselves in a variety of important ways. One of the biggest risks is postpartum depression. Women with untreated or undertreated bipolar disorders are at the greatest risk for postpartum depression. Bipolar postpartum depressions are often severe, and they are the most difficult bipolar depressions to treat. Postpartum psychosis is a serious and at times life-threatening complication mostly associated with bipolar I disorder. Preventing postpartum psychosis is paramount in women who may be at risk.

Being well before pregnancy is thought to mitigate many of the risks associated with bipolar disorder during pregnancy and is preventative to postpartum depression and postpartum psychosis. There has been no formal research on this topic.

We do not have an understanding of the myriad of effects that stress hormones have on gestating babies of undertreated or nontreated women with bipolar disorders.

A large Swedish population study of 320 treated and 554 untreated female patients with a bipolar disorder evaluated the effects of being treated vs. untreated during pregnancy. The comparison group was 332,137 nonbipolar women who had undergone pregnancy and delivery. The odds ratio (OR) of caesarean births for untreated women was 1.45. The OR for treated women was 1.56. Untreated women tended to bear small-for-gestational-age babies, and treated women had fewer small-for-gestational-age babies (OR 0.93). Untreated women were more likely to need to have labor induced (OR 2.12) compared with treated women (OR 1.57). Women with treated or untreated bipolar disorder have increased odds of premature delivery—delivery at less than thirty-seven weeks of gestation (OR 1.5). The study was not able to discern if untreated women were more or less seriously ill, nor was it able to discern the impact of individual medications. The results of this study do not show any impact of mood stabilizers. Adherence was measured by filling the prescribed medication (Bodén et al., 2012).

Many medications used to treat bipolar disorder pose a known risk for congenital problems. A significant problem is the lack of knowledge about many of the other treatments used to treat bipolar disorders.

There is one study that shows that high normal T4 levels in the first trimester have an increased risk of small size for gestational-age newborns, with an (OR 1.09) (Abonowara et al., 2012). This has not been replicated, and even if it is true for the general population, it may not apply to women taking HDT for affective illnesses.

Pregnancy's Normal Changes in Thyroid Functions

Pregnancy has a profound impact on the thyroid function. The thyroid gland increases 10% in size with iodine-sufficient diets and even more with iodine-insufficient diets. Production of T3 and T4 increase by 50%. The upper limit of TSH in pregnancy is now considered 2.3–2.5 mIU/L (Krhin and Besic, 2012; Stagnaro-Green et al., 2011).

HDT Treatment during Pregnancy

Despite the changes in the thyroid gland during pregnancy discussed above, patients on previously adequate doses of HDT rarely need an increase of T3. This is based on clinical impression only. There is no research to guide us. Nonetheless, if mood symptoms do reappear, T3 should be increased 12.5 mcg every five to seven days, watching for improvement or side effects.

Breastfeeding

Discussions about breastfeeding should take place at the first appointment after the patient is confirmed to be pregnant—or better yet, even before the patient is pregnant. Pregnant women inevitably encounter strong advocates for breastfeeding. However, the advocates have no ability to perform a risk-benefit analysis. Most advocates are so enthusiastic about breastfeeding that patients will feel great guilt if they don't breastfeed. In general, it is recommended that women with a bipolar disorder not breastfeed due to the destabilizing effects of sleep disruption. Most women, despite the risk for destabilization, elect to breastfeed. It is thought that women suffering a bipolar disorder need a block of six hours of uninterrupted sleep. With this six-hour block of sleep, naps can make up for the rest of needed sleep.

While the American Thyroid Association as well as the Endocrine Society recommend that women being treated with HDT to prevent the return of thyroid cancer continue HDT during pregnancy, both are completely silent about HDT and breastfeeding.

The literature is sparse on how much thyroid hormone passes into breast milk. There is some information that very little T4 is passed into breast milk. T3 also passes into milk in low amounts but more than T4.

The best recommendations for women taking HDT and breast feeding are:
1. First check mother's T4 and T3 levels. TSH levels are irrelevant in this situation. Despite low TSH and fairly high doses of thyroid hormones, T3 and or T4 levels can be normal or only slightly elevated. If this is the case, no adjustment need be made. Breastfeeding is safe.
2. If T3 and/or T4 are significantly high, then the safest route is to have the pediatrician check the infant's thyroid levels. If the infant's thyroid levels are high, then there are four alternatives.
    a. Timing may reduce levels in breastfed babies. Breastfeed immediately prior to taking thyroid dose. Avoid breastfeeding for the first four to six hours after taking T3. TMAX (time to reach maximal blood level) for T3 is one to two hours. For T4, it is 1.8 to 2.9 hours.
    b. Taper the thyroid dose to the point that the infant's thyroid levels normalize. Most of the time, patients will relapse into a deep depression.
    c. Stop breastfeeding.
    d. The middle ground is to continue breastfeeding and supplement with enough formula to reduce the infant's thyroid levels to normal.

Chapter 11: T3 vs. T4

To T3 or not to T3. That is the question.

–If Shakespeare had been a psychiatrist

In short: All the available preparations of thyroid hormone appear to work well. T3 has some practical and theoretical advantages over T4.

What is best: T3, T4, Armour Thyroid, Westhroid (or similar products made from animal thyroid), or a combination of T3 and T4?

There is no research directly comparing the outcome of one form of thyroid over the others in bipolar disorders. When thyroid hormones were originally synthesized and became commercially available, T4 was preferred due to its ease of measurement and low cost. Clinically, the results appear to be the same regardless of which thyroid-hormone preparation is used. There are practical and theoretic reasons to prefer T3 over T4, and they are discussed below. Each approach has its champions. The T3 proponents say that T3 is the most widely researched, and the T4 camp claims the same. Endocrinologists prefer T4 for replacement.

This author prefers T3. Dr. Michael Bauer, the world's foremost researcher of HDT, prefers T4. This may be because T4 is more available in Germany than T3 is. With regard to using a combination of T3 and T4, the literature contains research only about replacement therapy for hypothyroid patients. The commercially available preparations that were used contain a proportionately small amount of T3 and a larger amount of T4. This research gives us little guidance for HDT therapy. There are practical reasons, "medical reasons," and theoretical reasons to choose one approach over another. Keep in mind that for most patients, improvement with HDT is usually not gradual—it is not a rheostat, if you will; it is more like a light switch. Usually, no effect is seen until the dose that gives maximum benefit is reached, though, at times, at a dose just below the dose needed for maximum benefit an occasional patient will show some minimal improvement. For example, if a patient needs 125 mcg to get maximum benefit, minimal effects might be seen at 100 or 112.5 mcg.

Arguments for Using T3 Alone

1. **Patient pressure and expectation**. Reaching a therapeutic dose is faster with T3. There is always pressure to achieve improvement as fast as possible. Even when using T3, it is not uncommon for patients to become impatient with the wait. It is very tempting to increase the dose faster with a suicidal patient or a patient whose job is hanging in the balance. Increasing the dose faster than waiting the five half-lives it takes to reach the full blood level risks developing side effects. T3 is far more practical to use due to the shorter half-life of 24 hours compared with T4's half-life of seven days. The dose of T3 can be increased every five days, though in clinical practice, it is easier to see, evaluate, and change the dose weekly, if pressed for time. Most patients start to respond anywhere from 50 to 125 mcg. T4 patients will start to respond between 200 and 500 mcg. Some patients respond to a dose lower than 50 mcg; a few need doses higher than 125 mcg. This means that reaching a good blood level can be achieved significantly faster with T3. For example, if a patient's therapeutic dose of T3 is 125 mcg, it can be reached in 25 days as opposed to the equivalent dose of 500 mcg of T4 that would take 25 weeks.

    Increasing any treatment faster than five half-lives* increases the risks of overshooting the correct dose and getting into a toxic range. (It takes five half-lives to achieve steady state, after starting, increasing, or decreasing a dose of medicine.) This affects T4 more so than T3. With T4, the temptation is to push up the dose every three weeks (three half-lives achieves 85–90% of blood levels achieved at five half-lives).

2. **It maximizes the chance that a side effect will be detected and associated with a dose increase.** Correlating a side effect is much easier for both the prescriber and the patient if the side effect occurs within five days of increasing T3. For T4, a side effect may not show for five weeks. Clinical experience suggests that many patients, no matter how well prepared, will fail to connect a side effect to an increase in T4 dose that occurred five weeks earlier. Spending time with patients to educate them about potential side effects is always in order and can minimize the risk of missing an important side effect. Not all patients will listen or can concentrate long enough to learn and retain the information. Some patents will not want to know about side effects for fear that they will develop a side effect just because they fear it will happen. It is not unusual for patients to consult another physician because they have not recognized that they are experiencing a late-onset side effect. Not only can the patient incur the cost of an expensive work-up, but the primary care provider will order thyroid levels that inevitably will be high and tell the patient to discontinue all thyroid hormone. The patient, who is already hopeless from his or her depression, is now even more discouraged with HDT treatment and treatment in general. If this scenario happens with T3, patients will experience a relapse of symptoms within five days and remember my standard admonition to call if their mood is worsening.

3. **Resolution of side effects.** When side effects do occur, they will resolve faster with T3 than with T4. In general, with dose reduction, T3 side effects will improve in a day and will be gone within three days. It can take longer with T4—possibly a week until improvement and three weeks until resolution.

4. **Reverse T3.** Reverse T3 can be a problem when using T4. T4 is metabolized into T3 and reverse T3. Reverse T3 is biologically inactive. Any physiologic or even psychological stressor causes the body to shunt a greater proportion of T4 to reverse T3. The physiologic stressor can be most illnesses,

an infection, a surgery, an injury, or even an upper respiratory infection. There are a myriad of medical possibilities. Since patients suffering with a bipolar illness are frequently (perhaps constantly is more accurate) feeling stressed, they will be shunting T4 to reverse T3 just at a time when they need good thyroid levels. One wonders if this is the reason or a possible contributing reason why many bipolar relapses are associated with stressors. This does not happen with T3. So, using all T4 theoretically places patients at risk for a significant reduction in their thyroid levels just when they are stressed and need adequate thyroid levels the most. Since bipolar patients are easily and frequently stressed, T3 may be more protective.

5. **Converting T4 into T3**. Though it is rare, there are patients who have difficulties metabolizing T4 into T3.
6. **Compliance**. T4 is difficult for many patients to take. T4 must be taken one to two hours before a meal or two hours after a meal. Some pharmacy instructions state that T4 is not to be taken four hours before or after food. T3 absorption is minimally altered with concomitant food intake.
7. **Food**. T4 absorption has far more variability than T3. T4 should not be given to patients who find it difficult to stick to taking T4 one to two hours before or after food ingestion. Pharmacists will sometimes incorrectly give this recommendation with T3. The following has been clinically observed on at least two occasions: patients who had been stabilized on T4, taking their dose with breakfast, realized that they should be taking T4 two hours before or after breakfast. When the patient moved the T4 dose away from mealtime, more T4 was absorbed, leading to thyrotoxicosis. Alternatively, patients will get tired of taking T4 two hours before or after breakfast and will relapse, either because they've missed too many doses of T4 or because they've stopped altogether out of frustration with the dosing requirements.
8. **A number of drugs interfere with absorption of T4**. Antacids containing aluminum or magnesium, simethicone bile acid sequestrants (e.g., cholestyramine or colestipol), calcium carbonate, cation exchange resins (e.g., Kayexalate),

ferrous sulfate, orlistat, or sucralfate will also interfere with T3 but to a much lesser degree.
9. **First pass effects**. The first pass affects T4 to a far greater degree than T3. This makes dosage adjustments easier in the face of liver enzyme inducing medications (e.g., carbamazepine).
10. **Consistency of T4 between generics**. Cytomel (T3), is usually made by one company, so potency is consistent. Over the years, a generic company produced T3, only to give it up after a year or two. T4 is made by a number of companies, so patients will experience switching generics as insurance companies negotiate price breaks from one generic company or another. Over the years, inconsistencies in generic potencies have led many endocrinologists to prescribe Synthroid only.
11. **T3 may be healthier**. T3 may be healthier, at least in some respects. In a study of hypothyroid patients, T3 was substituted for equivalent doses of T4. Patients saw statistically mean improvement in the following areas: a weight loss of 4.6 pounds, a decrease in total cholesterol of 22.0 mg/dl, a decrease in non-HDL cholesterol of 16.5 mg/d, and a decrease in low-density lipoprotein-cholesterol of 16.4 mg/dl. This was without an appreciable change in heart rate, blood pressure, exercise tolerance, or insulin levels (Celi et al., 2011).
12. **Crossing cell membranes**. It is easier for T3 than for T4 to passively cross cell membranes.
13. **If using lithium**. Lithium interferes with the conversion of T4 to T3 in the brain and alters the structure of thyroglobulin (Chakrabarti, 2011). This could be a problem, especially when changing the lithium dose. Using only T3 bypasses this problem.

Arguments for Using T4

1. **Expense**. T4 is significantly less expensive than T3. This may be misleading. T4 certainly is less expensive than T3. However, since finding the right dose will usually take much longer, using T4 exposes the patient to a prolonged period of

symptoms or worse, waiting a longer time to find out that it isn't going to work. The longer it takes to see improvement, the more likely the patient will quit the thyroid trial or treatment altogether out of frustration.
2. **Easier to defend**. It is somewhat easier to defend the use of T4 than T3 to other physicians. Most physicians are taught to use T4 only. This is a poor reason.
3. **Advantage of a longer half-life**. There can be an advantage to a much longer half-life. Occasionally, T3 must be given twice a day. Dosing T4 twice a day is rarely needed. At least in theory, a more consistent blood level of thyroid hormone is closer to what the body experiences. How important a consistent blood level is has yet to be determined. Keep in mind that much of T4 will be changed to T3 (or reverse T3) on first pass effect, negating, at least to a certain degree, the advantages of T4.
4. **T3 shortages**. Occasionally, there are shortages of T3. The last was over nine years ago. These shortages have been short-lived—at most, a month—and can be bridged with T4.

Reasons to Use or Not Use Amour Thyroid, Nature Throid, Westhroid, or Similar Products

This includes compounded combinations of T3 and T4. These products are T3 and T4 in a ratio of 1 to 4.2. At these ratios, the problems are similar to using T4 alone.

1. The main reason to use these products is patient preference.
2. These products are more expensive than T4 or T3.
3. Over the years, problems with consistency of potency of these products have required recalls.
4. These have all the same problems as T4.

The Theoretical Winner

The theoretical winner is a combination of T3 and T4, weighted toward the larger portion being T3 for the following reasons:
1. Fetuses may need T4. See discussion of HDT in pregnancy.
2. There is some concern that some compartments of the body will have less-than-normal concentrations of thyroid

hormone if all of one type is used. A study of rats given subdermal T4 only did not provide adequate T3 levels to all tissues. Plasma TSH, T4, and T3 levels and 10 different tissue levels of T4 and T3 were measured after a 12–13 days of T4 infusion. This resulted in adequate tissue T3 levels in brown adipose tissue, cerebellum, cortex, and a few other tissue types. Most tissue showed a lower-than-normal T3 level. This suggests that the use of T4 therapy alone may not achieve normal T3 levels in all tissues. The authors of this study conclude, "It is evident that neither plasma T4 nor plasma T3 alone permit the prediction of the degree of change in T4 and T3 concentrations in tissues…The current replacement therapy of hypothyroidism [giving T4] should no longer be considered adequate"(Escobar-Morreale et al., 1995).

While a combination of T3 and T4 is the theoretical winner, there is no single compound that fulfills the criteria of mostly T3 with some T4

The Overall Winning Thyroid Preparation

The best type of thyroid preparation to use is whatever the patient is willing to take. For women with the potential to get pregnant, it is 150 mcg of T4 with the rest given as T3, titrating to maximum symptom relief or until side effects appear. The practical advantages of T3 make T3 the clear winner. In my experience, far fewer patients will quit a thyroid trial of T3 than T4. The overwhelming theoretical advantages along with the practical advantages argue for T3.

Chapter 12: Unique Aspects of HDT

I have never let my schooling interfere with my education.

–Mark Twain

In order to save the village, we had to destroy it.

–Unknown American officer after the city of Bến Tre, South Vietnam, was destroyed by allied bombing, February 7, 1968

In summary: HDT is unique among medications used to treat bipolar disorders. It is well tolerated, does not cause weight gain, helps cognition, and boosts energy. It may decrease medical morbidity and mortality of the bipolar disorders.

The emphasis in treating bipolar disorder is on controlling symptoms. Only recently has there been much discussion of preserving or improving functionality. While certainly welcoming symptom relief, most patients place returning to normal functioning very high on the list of what they wish for. How often do we watch patients slide down the socioeconomic ladder, many into disability? Loss of functionality often leads to job loss, bankruptcy, divorce, and almost universally decreases patients' self-esteem. Functional impairments can lead directly and indirectly to noncompliance with treatment. If the patient can't remember to go to appointments or take his or her medications, compliance is an issue. Patients will stop their medications in order to improve their functionality—that is, improved energy, improved cognition, and improvements in other functional impairments caused by the medications. Many would trade less control of symptoms for improved functionality. Restoring or improving functionality is often key to socioeconomic success.

Clarifying Clinical Impression vs. Clinical Observations

This chapter is based largely on a systematic evaluation of clinical observations. Note that there is a difference between clinical observation and clinical impression. Clinical impression is a preliminary observation based on a small number of patients. By definition, these observations have not been systematically evaluated. Treatment decisions based on clinical impressions should be limited to situations where all other more valid treatments have failed. In other words, they should be extremely rare. Still, even clinical impressions are not totally void of scientific merit. Where would we be today if John Cade's experience with lithium treatment of 10 manic patients been dismissed as a clinical impression? Clinical impressions should be considered an invitation for more careful observation and evaluation.

Clinical observation is defined as experiences with a medication with a minimum of 100 patients. In this case, the clinical observations are based on experiences of over 1,500 trials of thyroid treatment over the years. The great majority of trials of thyroid hormone were with high doses. To be certain, not all trials were successful. This author has published a number of studies based on the systematic evaluation of clinical observations, though not all are of HDT (Kelly, 2008; Kelly et al., 2013; Kelly and Lieberman, 2009; Kelly and Lieberman, 2017).

When compared with most medications used to treat the bipolar disorders, there are five features of HDT that make it unique: tolerability, lack of weight gain, improvement in cognition, improved energy, and improvement in patients' level of functioning.

Well Tolerated

Unlike so many of the medications used to treat bipolar disorder HDT is well tolerated. This has been remarked on in numerous studies (Bauer et al., 2003; Bauer et al., 2002; Bauer et al., 2015; Bauer et al., 2005; Bauer and Whybrow, 2001; Bauer and Whybrow, 1990; Kelly and Lieberman, 2009; Ricken et al., 2012a). In a particularly interesting experiment discussed in detail in chapter 13, when patients and controls were given a daily dose of 500 mcg of T4, 38% of normal control subjects (without affective illness) dropped out of treatment due to side effects, while none of the refractory patients suffering a major depression or bipolar depression dropped out, and they experienced great improvement (Bauer et al., 2002). This is not to say that thyrotoxic side effects are not possible;

it only indicates that the vast majority of bipolar patients do not experience thyrotoxic symptoms. If thyrotoxic symptoms happen, they can be easily handled by decreasing the dose of HDT.

Lack of Weight Gain/Increased Appetite

HDT appears to be weight neutral, but an occasional obese patient can experience profound weight loss. Interestingly, it is not unusual for HDT to increase appetite without weight gain. How? It would only be speculation, but the likely mechanism of action for this is through correcting for cellular hypothyroidism. When patients do lose weight, they experience a period of time when food is less interesting. Occasionally, patients will be concerned about this. You can reassure patients that once they reach their body's new (lower) set point, they will stop losing weight, and their interest in food will return.

Improved Energy

Most but not all patients receiving benefit from HDT will experience a normalization of their energy levels or at least a great improvement.

Improved Functioning

Many of our medications, while helping control symptoms, cause functional problems (destroy the village in order to save it). Yes, quetiapine can help bipolar depression, but most patients have major difficulties with sedation—at the very least in the morning, if not all day. Most patients believe that returning to a higher level of functioning is as important as symptom relief. Keeping a job, keeping a family intact, and being able to function well cognitively are of paramount importance to patients and families. HDT can and often does restore functioning to patients (Bauer and Whybrow, 1990). Cognition improvement is where HDT can be of greatest benefit. HDT is also helpful for the lassitude of depression. This can indirectly help cognition. Wanting to learn is often as important as the ability to learn.

Cognition: Author's Darwinist Observation

The bipolar disorders alone can cause cognitive problems (Green, 2006). We then compound the problem by adding medications that can cause cognitive problems in their own right and reduce functionality in other ways—for example, medications that worsen energy level and sedation. HDT does not harm cognition. In fact, most patients receive considerable benefit toward restoring cognition. Specifically, it can help best with word finding, name finding, fact-finding, and other manifestations of longer-term concentration that patients mistakenly refer to as memory problems. Clinically, the discovery that HDT can be of great benefit for cognition is based on a Darwinistic experience. Two studies have been published that show the usefulness of donepezil for treating the cognitive problems associated with bipolar disorders (Jacobsen and Comas-Díaz, 1999; Kelly, 2008). Both studies were case series that demonstrated that donepezil is often helpful for the cognitive problems of bipolar II and NOS patients. Both studies showed that bipolar I patients were not helped or were driven into mania (Jacobsen and Comas-Díaz, 1999; Kelly, 2008).

For a while, this author extensively used donepezil to treat bipolar II and NOS cognitive problems. When the 2013 edition of the Canadian bipolar treatment guidelines were published (Yatham et al., 2013), this author realized that the use of donepezil had been supplanted by HDT. It was at that time we realized that when HDT was used, donepezil was no longer needed. In other words, patients on HDT experience improvement—and in many cases, resolution—of cognition problems, so donepezil was simply no longer required. In addition, HDT can be used for both bipolar I, II, and NOS without causing mania. It should be kept in mind that HDT does not resolve every cognitive problem. At times, adjustment to medications that cause cognitive problems is still necessary—for example, lowering doses of valproic acid, lithium, and topiramate, to name a few.

Clinically, HDT is helpful for cognition for the following reasons:

1. The observation of cognition improvement with HDT in more than 500 patients with bipolar disorder.

2. Many patients and patients' families specifically remarked about cognitive improvement with HDT treatment. The cognitive effects are enduring as long as one takes an adequate thyroid dose.
3. Objective feedback based on improved job performance or improved grades indicated cognitive improvement.
4. Neuroimaging studies show that HDT specifically helps with brain functioning. (See chapter 5.)

Most but not all patients experience cognitive improvement. In general, HDT helps other symptoms; it usually helps cognition. Patients with relatively intact cognition rarely show improvement, and only a small percentage of patients with poor cognition have failed to show much if any improvement.

It could be argued that the basis of improved cognition was due to improvement of bipolar symptoms in general. Likely, there are elements of both the resolution of depression and specific effects of HDT that are helpful to cognition. Since there are no formal studies of HDT and cognition, the above observations that HDT is helpful for cognition must be viewed with some skepticism.

Chapter 13: The Theory of How Thyroid Hormone Works in Treatment of Bipolar Disorders

Science is founded on uncertainty. Each time we learn something new and surprising, the astonishment comes with the realization that we were wrong before.
–Lewis Thomas

Summary: HDT may work by correcting cellular hypothyroidism.

A hypothesis of the mechanism of action of HDT is that HDT corrects for cellular hypothyroidism. Clearly, HDT is exerting some type of influence on patients who improve or become euthymic. Does HDT act the way "cold medications" do? That is, do they only give symptomatic relief, or does HDT have some unique effects that correct an underlying physiologic deficit?

The evidence strongly points to HDT correcting an underlying physiologic defect. Our hypothesis is that treatment with HDT results in the correction of cellular hypothyroidism. The cellular hypothyroidism is caused by difficulties in getting thyroid hormone across cell membranes due to a shortage of adenosine 5'-triphosphate (ATP). Getting thyroid hormone into cells is energy intensive and dependent on ATP levels. ATP is produced in the mitochondria. The shortage of ATP is the direct result of mitochondrial defects found in the bipolar disorders. The high circulating levels of thyroid hormone are sufficient to drive enough thyroid hormones into cells to overcome the deficiency caused by the decreased ATP levels (Kelly, 2016).

What Research Supports the Hypothesis?

There are numerous studies showing that HDT can greatly improve symptoms of bipolar depression, often to the point of lasting euthymia (Bauer et al., 2003; Bauer et al., 2002; Bauer et al., 2015; Bauer et al., 2005; Bauer and Whybrow, 2001; Bauer and Whybrow, 1990; Kelly and Lieberman, 2009; Ricken et al., 2012a). The effectiveness of HDT is reflected by its inclusion in multiple bipolar treatment guidelines (Crismon et al., 2007; Hirschfeld, 2010; Sachs et al., 2000; Yatham et al., 2013).

As discussed in chapter 4, two FDG-PET studies show that many of the numerous areas of the brain are in a hypermetabolic state that is corrected with HDT. Both studies show normalization of the hypermetabolic areas of the brain known to be involved in depression, and this down regulation in neurophysiology directly correlates with symptom improvement, thus showing that HDT has a "normalizing" effect on the brain (Bauer et al., 2005) (Bauer et al., 2015).

Thyroid Hormone Is Well Tolerated

As discussed in chapter 12, HDT is remarkably well tolerated for individuals suffering from a bipolar disorder (Bauer et al., 2003; Bauer et al., 2002; Bauer et al., 2015; Bauer et al., 2005; Bauer and Whybrow, 2001; Bauer and Whybrow, 1990; Kelly and Lieberman, 2009; Ricken et al., 2012a). Yet, as previously discussed, in euthyroid nonaffectively ill individuals, HDT does not produce euphoria or increased energy; it just causes side effects (Bauer et al., 2002). The contrast between the reactions of these two groups goes far in supporting the hypothesis.

Mitochondria Dysfunction

Mitochondria produce ATP, which provides 95% of cells' energy needs. Patients with mitochondrial disorders have symptoms similar to affective disorders (Higashiguchi et al., 2009; Rezin et al., 2009). There is a consensus that mitochondrial dysfunction plays a key role in bipolar (Manji et al., 2012; Stork and Renshaw, 2005).

These studies suggest that cellular bioenergetics play a role in bipolar disorders and that HDT treatment can significantly impact both symptoms and neurophysiology.

Evidence of Low ATP Levels

Multiple functional MRI studies have shown decreased pH, phosphocreatine, and ATP levels as well as increased lactate levels in the brain regions associated with the bipolar disorders. These are hallmarks of decreased energy metabolism (Hennemann et al., 2001; Jou et al., 2009; Stork and Renshaw, 2005; Sun et al., 2006).

These studies suggest that cellular bioenergetics play a role in bipolar disorders and that HDT treatment can significantly impact both symptoms and neurophysiology.

Thyroid Hormone Transportation

Previously, it was thought that thyroid hormones passively diffused into cells. We now understand that thyroid transportation is energy intensive. Multiple studies have shown that thyroid hormone uptake with human tissues is ATP dependent, and low ATP can limit metabolism. Even small changes in ATP levels lower intracellular T3 levels. This has been established in vitro and in vivo in rats (Hennemann et al., 2001). Gergő Tóth and his group state, "It is now widely accepted that the cellular uptake of THs is effected by energy dependent, carrier-mediated processes" (Tóth et al., 2013). Other research and a review article support these conclusions (Dietrich et al., 2008; Hennemann et al., 2001; Holtorf, 2014).

Thyroid Hormone in the Pituitary

If low ATP levels result in the decreased transportation of T3 and T4, why does this not cause overt hypothyroidism? It turns out that the pituitary uses different thyroid hormone transmitters than found in peripheral tissues (Everts et al., 1996; Hennemann et al., 2001; Köhrle, 2007; Wassen et al., 2000).

It has previously been established that cellular thyroid levels can be low despite normal thyroid pituitary and blood levels. Under certain conditions, it is a normal physiological response (e.g., starvation). A 1986 review paper cited many lines of experimental evidence that T3 levels can be low in peripheral tissues yet normal in the pituitary (van der Heyden et al., 1986). At least 10 different, energy-dependent thyroid hormone transporters have been identified in humans, and under normal circumstances, "They guarantee that intracellular levels of THs are higher than in blood plasma or interstitial fluids" (Dietrich et al., 2008). Entry of the thyroid hormone into the pituitary is not energy dependent. Thus, if the energy-dependent thyroid hormone transporters are disrupted, intercellular thyroid hormone levels suffer. This conclusion is based on human studies and animal studies, both in vivo and in vitro. The lines of research included: fasting states; nonthyroidal illnesses; and three different medications—amiodarone, benzodiazepines, and SKF

L-94901 (an experimental medication)—that disturb the entry of thyroid hormones into cells (Everts et al., 1996). The pituitary regulates thyroid hormone production based on T3 and T4 blood levels. The pituitary thyroid levels are not dependent on active transportation and therefore reflect serum levels of thyroid hormone found in the blood, not in cells. In the bipolar disorders, the pituitary "reads" normal thyroid blood levels even while the rest of the body is suffering from cellular hypothyroidism.

Three Coincidences That May Not Be Coincidences

The First Coincidence: Depression or Hypothyroidism

There is considerable overlap between depressive symptoms and hypothyroid symptoms. Hypothyroid symptoms include weakness, sleepiness, lethargy, fatigue, weight gain, menstrual disruption, slow movement, depression, anorexia, muscle pains, joint pains, constipation, memory difficulties, low attention span, slow calculations, lack of enthusiasm, anxiety, and irritability (Monaco, 2003). According to the DSM-IV and DSM-IV-TR, depression symptoms and hypothyroid symptoms are so similar that hypothyroidism must be ruled out before a diagnosis of major depression can be given.

Clinically, it is not unusual for depressed patients prior to HDT treatments to suspect that they are suffering from hypothyroidism. This is a greater problem than one would think. Many patients, in an effort to understand or find the cause of their symptoms, have studied signs and symptoms of hypothyroidism, some quite extensively. Many have concluded that they are hypothyroid. When they see their primary care doctor or an endocrinologist, they are told that their thyroid levels are normal. Most patients do not relate this until they feel better with HDT treatment. With HDT, these patients are no longer the coldest ones in the room. They are no longer in constant battle with their spouses over thermostat settings. It turns out that research actually backs up the phenomenon of patients feeling that their thyroid levels are inadequate, and the phenomenon is not limited to affectively ill individuals (Kalra and Khandelwal, 2011).

It should be noted that a lack of hypothyroid symptoms except for depression does not appear to decrease the chance of successful treatment with HDT. Systematic evaluation may clarify this issue.

Hypothyroid patients have similar experiences. Many feel they are not on enough thyroid hormone. They complain of feeling dull and express other hypothyroid symptoms, only to be told that their thyroid levels are fine (Kalra and Khandelwal, 2011).

The Second Coincidence: Overlap of the Mortality and Morbidity of Hypothyroidism and the Bipolar Disorders

Another remarkable coincidence is the substantial overlap between the medical sequelae of hypothyroidism and bipolar disorders. Both are associated with vitamin D deficiency, diabetes mellitus, depression, hypertension, and heart disease (Kalra and Khandelwal, 2011; Leboyer et al., 2012).

Patients with a bipolar disorder suffer premature death—on average, 10 to 20 years earlier than the general public (Leboyer et al., 2012). This is primarily from medical causes. Suicide, by comparison, plays a much smaller role in the premature death of our patients (Laursen, 2011; Leboyer et al., 2012). The premature death in the bipolar disorders has been attributed to a lower socioeconomic status or poor lifestyle, such as poor diet, obesity, poor medical care, and use of drugs and alcohol. However, there is more to this than lack of self-care. It is possible that cellular hypothyroidism plays a role in the premature death, paralleling the effects of hypothyroidism.

The Third Coincidence: Thyrotoxic Symptoms Are Associated with Intercellular Levels of Thyroid Hormone

Even in hyperthyroidism, it has long been known that there is a disconnect between symptoms and thyroid levels. In hyperthyroidism, the levels of T3 and T4 are only moderately correlated with thyrotoxic symptoms (Bahn et al., 2011). The symptoms are correlated with cellular levels of thyroid hormones (Kalra and Khandelwal, 2011).

Other Supportive Evidence

The theory rests on the supposition that cellular hypothyroidism is present. Unfortunately, as yet, there is no direct way to measure cellular thyroid levels in humans. Intracellular thyroid levels in animals are determined by sacrificing the animal (Kalra and Khandelwal, 2011).

There is sufficient evidence to support the theory that HDT's mechanism of action is correcting cellular hypothyroidism. The brain has the highest concentration of mitochondria and the highest metabolic activity of the body (Bauer et al., 2015; Bauer et al., 2005; Holtorf, 2014) so it is no surprise that even mildly low ATP can have profound effects. As shown by FDG-PET imaging studies, HDT treatment can reverse overactivity in brain regions that are involved in bipolar depression while significantly reducing bipolar depressive symptoms (Bauer et al., 2015; Bauer et al., 2005).

The evidence connecting bipolar disorders with mitochondrial dysfunction also indicates an association with low ATP levels (Higashiguchi et al., 2009; Rezin et al., 2009). There is evidence that the pituitary thyroid hormone transport system is different than the rest of the body. The pituitary is less energy dependent, compared with the rest of the body. This leads to normal pituitary levels and normal blood of levels of thyroid hormone, even though the rest of the body is experiencing cellular hypothyroidism (Kelly, 2016).

There are intriguing implications and ramifications of this theory:

1. The single most important implication is that a cellular hypothyroid state could partially explain part of the pathophysiology of bipolar disorders.
2. The theory, if true, would mean that HDT would, by correcting for cellular hypothyroidism, decrease the medical morbidity and mortality associated with the bipolar disorders. Potentially, this could be a leap forward in the treatment of bipolar disorders, giving us for the first time a treatment that not only can help control the symptoms of bipolar disorder but also decrease the medical morbidity and mortality associated with bipolar disorders.

3. There is a link between suicide attempts and thyroid-axis disturbance (Duval et al., 2010). It is possible that correcting cellular hypothyroidism will decrease the suicide rate beyond that found with symptom relief.
4. The theory, if correct, reinforces the research showing that HDT is a relatively safe treatment.
5. The theory, if correct, would explain why HDT is so well tolerated in patients with bipolar disorders, even though the same high doses in nonaffectively ill individuals cause thyrotoxicity.
6. Despite the widely held suspicion that a defect in the thyroid axis plays a role in bipolar disorders, the defect has never been found. This relationship has been the subject of much research, yet an exact link has been elusive (Chakrabarti, 2011). This theory gives a plausible explanation of this long-sought "missing link." Plainly, if cellular hypothyroidism already exists, any further disturbance of the HPT axis would have a disproportionate effect and more likely be found.
7. If the theory is correct, it would increase our understanding of the role of low intercellular ATP levels and the mitochondrial dysfunction found in the bipolar disorders.
8. If the theory is correct, blood levels of thyroid hormone in bipolar individuals would be useless in determining their thyroid status (except that low thyroid blood levels still indicate frank hypothyroidism).
9. If the theory is correct, using thyroid hormone levels to determine HDT treatment doses would be misleading and therefore irrelevant. Most patients who respond have significantly elevated thyroid hormones yet experience no side effects.
10. If the theory is correct, it would justify the clinical practice of determining HDT dosing by response. Response would be determined by increasing the dose of thyroid hormone until obtaining maximal symptom relief or the development of thyrotoxic symptoms. In general, thyrotoxic symptoms would indicate the need to decrease the dose.

11. If the theory is correct, it would challenge the long held belief that blood thyroid hormone measurements should be the sole determinant of thyroid dosing—not just in bipolar disorder but any time thyroid replacement is given.
12. Bipolar relapses are complex and multifactorial. Many relapses appear to be triggered by stress. Physical stress and/or psychological stress have been shown to shunt T4 to reverse T3 (Holtorf, 2014). Reverse T3 is biologically inactive. One possible explanation of why stress causes relapses or is a contributing factor to relapses could be the stress-induced shunting of T4 to reverse T3, which would further exacerbate the already existing cellular hypothyroid state.
13. Obesity is a tremendous problem among patients with a bipolar disorder. Correcting for cellular hypothyroidism could potentially cut the rate of obesity.
14. If the theory is correct, it further legitimizes HDT as a valid treatment for bipolar depression.
15. Since HDT does not universally help all patients suffering from a bipolar disorder, response to HDT may represent a biologic marker for a type of bipolar disorder that is not readily separated based on symptoms.

Weaknesses of Theory

The proposed theory may be overly simplistic. Thyroid transportation across the cell membrane is not fully understood. However, even if the theory is overly simplistic or parts are wrong, the theory could still be substantially correct and be useful.

The Theory Is Easily Tested

Once a method of measuring cellular levels of thyroid hormones is perfected, the theory can be easily tested.

End Thought

Thus, we come to a query posed earlier. That is, if the theory that HDT works by correcting cellular hypothyroidism is correct, the question is not "what are the risks of using HDT?" The question is "what are the risks of not using HDT?"

If we have a medication that not only improves the quality of patients' lives by decreasing or stopping bipolar symptoms, but it is also as safe or safer than most other medicines used for the bipolar disorders, improves cognition, and decreases the associated medical morbidity and mortality of the bipolar disorders, then the latter question is by far the most important question.

Chapter 14: Post Hoc Ergo Propter Hoc: Where the Field of Endocrinology Went Wrong

Selected Comments about Opposition to the Use of High-Dose Thyroid

Facts are stubborn things; and whatever may be our wishes, our inclinations, or the dictates of our passions, they cannot alter the state of facts and evidence.

–John Adams

In summary: The field of endocrinology has made the classic mistake that has so often plagued scientific endeavors—medicine, in particular. That is, it adopted a correlation as a causation. The medical sequelae of hyperthyroidism are not from high circulating levels of thyroid hormone. The sequelae of hyperthyroidism are likely due to an autoimmune process. Indeed, many of the sequelae have already been proven to be from an autoimmune process.

Why This Chapter and the Next?

This chapter and the next were the most difficult chapters in the book. The opposition to the use of HDT must be addressed. The opposition comes from physicians not familiar with the science and safety of HDT. Over the years, colleagues and friends have adopted the use of HDT with good results only to abandon HDT later under an onslaught of criticism. The following case study illustrates a case where another doctor directly interfered with a patient's care. The use of high-dose thyroid for the treatment of bipolar disorder has never been endorsed by endocrinologists and is considered dangerous (Rosenthal et al., 2011). If we are reticent to assert our knowledge and the evidence base—to tell the emperor that he is wearing no clothes—then our patients and their families will suffer. The successful use of HDT requires a thorough understanding of the science, lest the practitioner be buried by the ignorance of others. The information presented in this book stems from a decade of research and over 30 years of experience with thyroid hormones and dealing with others who sometimes strongly object to HDT.

Case vignette: BC is a 45 yo female sent for an endocrine consultation by her primary care doctor because of elevated T3 levels. The T3 levels were directly attributed to the use of high-dose T3. BC suffered from a severe bipolar II disorder that at one point had degenerated into a severe mixed-symptom depression. She had failed 22 trials of other medications which included Li, carbamazepine, clozapine and valproic acid. She had been fired from five jobs in the last three years and had alienated her friends and family. She was unable to obtain Social Security disability. All this led to a series of suicide attempts, the last and most serious, an overdose of acetaminophen and alcohol poisoning that came close to ending her life. T3 was added and titrated up. She became euthymic after the dose of 150 mcg of T3 was reached, added to 250 mg/d of lamotrigine, 375 mg/d of oxcarbazepine and 2.5 mg every other day of aripiprazole. She returned to work and had started winning back her friends and family. BK had no signs or symptoms of thyrotoxicity. She had been euthymic for a year and a half.

The endocrinologist diagnosed the patient with "iatrogenic hyperthyroidism" and warned the patient of dire cardiovascular and osteoporosis risks. The endocrinologist, without consultation, told the patient to immediately discontinue T3. The patient expressed concerns about what this would do to her depression. Despite these concerns, the endocrinologist insisted that she stop all of the T3. The endocrinologist did not instruct the patient to contact the prescribing psychiatrist, nor did the endocrinologist alert the prescribing psychiatrist that T3 was going to be discontinued. The patient complied and stopped all T3. Within three days, the patient said, "I plunged into the blackest depression I have ever experienced." She started giving away her possessions and had a detailed suicide plan. Alarmed, her family contacted the psychiatrist, and the T3 was resumed. Within a week she felt better, and by three weeks was again euthymic.

This endocrinologist's actions were suboptimal for a number of reasons:

1. The endocrinologist failed to do a proper risk-benefit analysis. Despite the patient voicing concern about a return of depression, the endocrinologist failed to query what a relapse of her bipolar disorder may mean and what risks this would pose for her. Even if the HDT posed the risk that the endocrinologist believed it did, the benefits of HDT for this patient far outweighed the risk.
2. There is a cardiac risk to abruptly stopping thyroid medication.
3. Labeling a patient's condition as hyperthyroid or "iatrogenic hyperthyroidism" does not fit the definition of hyperthyroidism. It fails in two important ways. First, the patient was not experiencing any thyrotoxic symptoms; and second, the source of the high circulating levels of thyroid hormone was external. The definition of hyperthyroidism requires the source of the thyroid hormone to be internal and requires the presence of thyrotoxic symptoms.
4. Changing a medication used to treat an illness outside one's area of expertise without contacting or notifying the prescribing physician is what? Dangerous, foolish, arrogant, rude, or asking for a malpractice suit. Pick one.
5. Even if the endocrinologists had been correct about the risks of high-dose thyroid, the risk-benefit ratio for this patient greatly favors the continuation of HDT.

Modern medicine is a team effort. The prescribing physician needs to know what the consulting physician is doing. Notifying the prescribing physician in this case could have avoided a severe, life-threatening bipolar relapse. Unfortunately, it is an all-too-common occurrence that other physicians advise patients to discontinue HDT without doing a risk-benefit analysis or talking to the prescribing physician. They discontinue HDT based on the myth that it is causing a hyperthyroid state and therefore poses a danger to the patient's health. As discussed in chapters 4, 6, and 7, HDT is as safe as or safer than most psychiatric medications. The question arises, How did we arrive at this state where the use of HDT is socially controversial but not scientifically controversial?

Post Hoc Ergo Propter Hoc

Medicine has a long history of post hoc ergo propter hoc errors. That is, mistaking correlations as causations. An example of this was the previously routine practice of treating postmenopausal women with estrogen replacement. It was believed that the estrogen replacement decreased heart disease and had other benefits. In the women observed, there was, in fact, less heart disease. When a more careful, longer, and larger observation study was conducted, estrogen replacement was shown to significantly increase mortality, chiefly through an increased risk of breast cancer. Worse, it didn't protect against heart disease. The original observation was true. The women given estrogen replacement did have less heart disease and lived longer than the general public. The problem was that the observation was made in women who had a good socioeconomic status, and these women typically have less cardiovascular disease and live longer than the general population.

Where the Field of Endocrinology Went Wrong

Reviewing the endocrinology literature reveals the belief that high circulating levels of thyroid hormone cause the medical sequela of hyperthyroidism. This was taught to us in medical school. This belief is firmly rooted, despite the large body of evidence to the contrary discussed earlier in this book. Interestingly, when discussing HDT, the literature does not adhere to the definitions of hyperthyroidism and thyrotoxicosis. A litany of errors that illustrate this point is discussed in the osteoporosis chapter and the cardiovascular chapter. It would appear that when research "confirms" expectations, it receives less scrutiny. Yet, we have seen that the few papers that continue to support the notion that high circulating levels of thyroid hormone cause problems fall apart when closely scrutinized.

Endocrinology has fallen into a trap of believing that the high circulating levels of thyroid hormone it is the cause of the medical sequelae of hyperthyroidism. To be fair, this was an easy assumption to make. After all, high thyroid levels cause thyrotoxic symptoms and increased levels of bone-turnover markers (see chapter 6). This was an especially easy assumption to make because of the lack of alternative etiologies.

Yet as shown in earlier chapters, a close and thorough review of the literature reveals that humans given HDT to treat bipolar disorder or to suppress the recurrence of thyroid cancer don't show the morbidity and mortality of hyperthyroidism, nor do they show significant bone loss. In the few prospective studies that kept track of mortality, there is a mathematical trend of fewer deaths of HDT-treated patients when compared with controls. (See chapter 7.) While the animal studies do show a decrease in bone density, the doses of thyroid hormone used were thousands of times larger than those used in human HDT studies. (See chapter 6.) Of particular interest, there is now an alternative etiology, discussed below, for the medical sequela of hyperthyroidism. It is an alternative etiology that has been proven to be true at least for some of the medical sequelae associated with hyperthyroidism.

How the Myth Perpetuates Itself

This is where Spinoza's quote from chapter 4 is prescient. "Many errors, of a truth, consist merely in the application of the wrong names of things." When discussing the use of HDT, endocrinologists almost universally fail to use the correct definition of hyperthyroidism and/or fail to use it properly. Despite the source of the thyroid hormones being external and regardless of the lack of signs and symptoms of thyrotoxicosis, endocrinologists will refer to HDT as subclinical hyperthyroidism, hyperthyroidism, or iatrogenic hyperthyroidism. This could be the single biggest reason why the myth is so persistent. In fact, in all the endocrine literature that was used to prepare this book, not one example could be found where HDT was not identified or mistaken as hyperthyroidism or subclinical hyperthyroidism in some fashion.

Key examples of this come from the American Thyroid Association and the British Thyroid Association Guidelines. In the first example, despite the lack of symptoms, the term "subclinical thyrotoxicosis" was used in the 2009 *Revised American Thyroid Association Management Guidelines for Patients with Thyroid Nodules and Differentiated Thyroid Cancer* (Cooper et al., 2009). In regard to the cardiovascular risks, the guidelines state the adverse risks "of TSH suppression may include the known consequences of subclinical thyrotoxicosis." Yet the only citation referred to was actually a study of subclinical hyperthyroidism (Sawin et al., 1994). The guidelines go on to assert that there is a risk of osteoporosis with HDT. However, while the study finds that hyperthyroidism is a risk for osteoporosis, curiously the citation used states, "The evidence that exogenous (thyroid) is a risk factor for osteoporosis is therefore inconclusive" (Toft, 2001).

The second key example of this comes from the British Thyroid Association's *Guidelines for the Management of Thyroid Cancer* (Perros et al., 2014). The guidelines cite three studies that purportedly show that HDT poses cardiovascular risks. However, when the citations are examined, two of the studies were of subclinical hyperthyroidism and therefore irrelevant. The third citation, the only one that did not include any form of hyperthyroidism, was the troubled Fujimoto study (see chapter 6). It is curious that both task forces responsible for the development of guidelines that involve the use of HDT to prevent the reoccurrence thyroid cancer failed to consider the extensive literature that directly examined the risks of external HDT. This falls below the standard that one expects from a panel of experts. One has to wonder how many endocrinologists, out of fear of hyperthyroid sequelae, minimize the dose of HDT used to suppress the return of thyroid cancer, thereby placing a patient at a greater risk for reoccurrence of thyroid cancer. How many patients taking HDT to prevent the return of thyroid cancer are noncompliant with treatment because they fear osteoporosis or heart disease?

This mistaking HDT for hyperthyroidism did not improve with the American Thyroid Association's most recent *Management Guidelines for Adult Patients with Thyroid Nodules and Differentiated Thyroid Cancer*, published in 2016 (Haugen et al., 2016). This guideline continues to abuse the definition of hyperthyroidism by continuing to consider HDT as "hyperthyroidism." They continue to cite studies that directly contradict their assertion that HDT is a risk factor for osteoporosis. They cite the Toft study, as discussed above, which directly contradicts their assertion. Surprisingly, they then double down on their error by including a new citation, Chen et al., which also contradicts their assertion. Chen et al. states, "Women with differentiated thyroid cancer who had long-term (mean, 7.3 +/- 3.0 years) T4 therapy and suppressed TSH levels had no evidence of lower BMD." The Chen et al. statement also includes postmenopausal women who showed no statistical difference between the group treated with HDT and the healthy control group (Chen et al., 2004).

Thyroid Blood Levels: Numbers Are Not Enough

The value of blood levels for determining adequacy of thyroid levels has been questioned since first utilized. First, "normal" thyroid laboratory values are based on large population studies. This does not rule out that there are individuals whose normal thyroid needs may be higher than "normal thyroid levels." Second, there is no allowance for illnesses that make it difficult for the thyroid hormone to cross cell membranes (laboratory measurements of thyroid levels are determined from serum). Third, the mechanism of action of thyroid hormones is intercellular, and blood levels don't always reflect intercellular levels. In untreated Graves' disease, the severity of symptoms is only loosely correlated with thyroid blood levels. As far back as 1989, it has been known that thyrotoxic symptoms correlate better with intracellular thyroid hormone levels than with blood levels (Trzepacz et al., 1989).

The American Association of Clinical Endocrinologists and the American Thyroid Association hypothyroid treatment guidelines recommend using TSH levels alone in determining thyroid dosing for hypothyroid patients (Garber et al., 2012). Yet there has always been a subgroup of endocrinologists that questions the value of managing hypothyroidism based on blood thyroid hormone levels alone. They believe clinical assessment of symptoms and the patient's sense of well-being should be considered in determining thyroid dosing. A survey of hypothyroid patients treated based on TSH levels alone revealed that they are often left with significant residual symptoms such as word-finding difficulty, concentration problems, memory problems, lack of energy, lethargy, weight gain, inability to think clearly, coordination problems, clumsiness, and aches and pains—all despite "normal" thyroid levels (Benvenga, 2013).

Research shows that patients with hypothyroidism prefer that their thyroid doses be determined by clinical assessment rather than TSH levels. When assessed clinically without TSH levels, patients on average received T4 doses that were 50 mcg higher than dosing based on TSH levels. When thyroid dosing was determined by well-being, the highest scores were obtained when the serum level of TSH was < 0.2 (Kalra and Khandelwal, 2011). Endocrinologists justify their rigid adherence to lab values practice based on the belief that high circulating levels of thyroid hormone cause the same medical sequela as hyperthyroidism. For psychiatrists and indeed for most physicians, it seems an unwise policy not to listen to patients and even worse to dismiss signs and symptoms of a disease as a matter of principle. Before the advent of thyroid blood testing, physicians had to dose thyroid hormones based solely on clinical findings, and the average dose of thyroid was higher.

An Inevitable Conclusion

The post hoc ergo propter hoc error that the sequela of hyperthyroidism is due to the high circulating levels of thyroid hormone has caused the field of endocrinology to fail to recognize that high circulating levels of thyroid hormone it is not the same as and is not the cause of the medical sequela associated with hyperthyroidism (Kelly, 2016). There is a fundamental disconnect between the safety of HDT as reviewed in the prior chapters and the myriad of medical complications associated with hyperthyroidism. Given the safety record of HDT and the high morbidity and mortality rate of hyperthyroidism, one is logically compelled to conclude that high circulating levels of thyroid hormones are not the cause of the major medical sequela of hyperthyroidism.

While it is beyond the scope of this book to make a definitive alternative argument, there is an attractive alternative etiology of the medical sequela of hyperthyroidism nonetheless.

The Alternative Etiology of the Medical Sequela of Hyperthyroidism

Why does hyperthyroidism cause osteoporosis and heart problems while HDT treatment does not? The most likely etiology of the medical sequela of hyperthyroidism is related to an autoimmune process. There is growing evidence that many or even all of the sequelae previously attributed to high circulating levels of thyroid hormone are due an autoimmune process (e.g., cardiovascular disease, pulmonary arterial hypertension, and myxomatous cardiac valve disease) (Biondi, 2012).

In areas where iodine is readily available in the diet, Graves' disease accounts for the great majority of hyperthyroid cases. Graves' disease is an autoimmune disease caused by TSH receptor (TSHr) antibodies. TSHr antibodies mimic TSH (Biondi and Kahaly, 2010) and stimulate TSH receptors, causing the high circulating levels of thyroid hormone in the absence of TSH (Bahn et al., 2011). This is the cause of the low TSH and high T3 and T4. Even though TSH antibodies mimic TSH, they do not show up in routine TSH screening. Thus, in Graves' disease, the thyroid gland is healthy.

Graves' disease effects are not limited to the thyroid gland; 90% of patients have one or more other pathologies. TSH receptors are not limited to the thyroid gland. Autoimmune antibodies are now fully accepted as the cause of exophthalmos (Wall and Lahooti, 2010) and Graves' pretibial myxedema (Topliss and Eastman, 2004). TSH receptors can be found in other tissues, including fat, fibroblasts, bone, brain, kidney, testis, heart, and cells of the immune system (Drvota et al., 1995; Gershengorn and Neumann, 2012). Toxic multinodular goiter has autoimmune components that are less well understood than those seen in Graves', but nonetheless, it has autoimmune aspects.

TSH receptor antibodies are not the only autoimmune process affecting patients with hyperthyroidism. Autoimmune disorders including Graves' as a rule are accompanied by other autoimmune problems (Biondi, 2012). For example, 27% of patients with rheumatoid arthritis also have an autoimmune thyroid disease (Benvenga, 2013). Graves' disease is linked with other autoimmune complications, including pernicious anemia, Addison's disease (Topliss and Eastman, 2004), pulmonary hypertension, heart valve dysfunction, and other cardiomyopathies (Biondi and Kahaly, 2010).

Autoimmune disorders are often linked to hyperthyroidism; for example, pulmonary hypertension is linked to hyperthyroidism and autoimmune diseases. A family or personal history of autoimmune thyroid disease is reported in roughly half of the patients with pulmonary arterial hypertension (Klein and Danzi, 2007). Unlike lithium, which can induce thyroid autoimmunity (Chakrabarti, 2011), there is no suspicion that HDT is associated with autoimmune problems.

One of the reasons that endocrinologists hold to the view that HDT is dangerous is that long-term follow-up of hyperthyroid patients shows an increased morbidity and mortality from higher doses of a thyroid replacement. But what they have failed to realize is that the autoimmune process often persists even after thyroid ablation. In fact, autoimmune problems can substantially worsen for a time after surgery. While most autoimmune problems improve with ablation of the thyroid gland, at least 10% of patients persist with autoimmune problems (Laurberg et al., 2008). The Belaya paper showing that bone loss continued for an average of 3.5 years after achieving normal thyroid levels supports the notion that a process other than high circulating levels of thyroid hormone is responsible for causing the medical problems associated with hyperthyroidism. It also shows that high circulating levels of thyroid hormone do not cause bone loss (Belaya et al., 2007). This is why using studies of subclinical hyperthyroidism or studies of patients on replacement doses of thyroid who previously had hyperthyroidism cannot be used as evidence for determining the safety of external HDT.

While ablating the thyroid gland seems to reduce thyroid antibodies over time, it seems a questionable practice to remove a perfectly healthy organ to address only one component of a complicated autoimmune process. More research into alternative treatments would seem to be in order.

Chapter 15: Psychiatrists' Role as Specialists

One half of what you were taught as medical students will in 10 years have been shown to be wrong, and the trouble is, your teachers don't know which half.

–C. Sidney Burwell (1893–1967) *British Medical Journal* 2, 113, 1956

...so the most important thing to learn is how to learn on your own.

-David Sackett, often referred to as the "father of evidence-based medicine" addition to
C. Sidney Burwell Statement

Endocrinologists Routinely Use HDT

When considering the use of HDT treatment for the bipolar disorders, keep in mind that endocrinologists routinely use HDT to prevent the return of thyroid cancer. The mortality of thyroid cancer, once the initial surgery has been performed and/or the thyroid gland has been ablated by radioiodine, is less than the mortality of the bipolar disorders. The morbidity of the bipolar disorders—that is, the suffering of individuals with bipolar disorder and the suffering of the family of an individual with bipolar disorder—is far greater than the morbidity associated with thyroid cancer.

If We Are to Practice Evidence-Based Medicine

Many of our patients are desperate for relief. If we are to present ourselves as specialists, if we truly want to help our patients, we must be willing to look beyond what is spoon-fed to us. If we are to practice evidence-based medicine, we need to pay particular attention to "orphan" medications—that is, medications that do not have the financial backing to be promoted yet have an evidence base. There is an ample database of evidence that HDT is both effective and safe, and there is supporting neuroimaging evidence. HDT is as safe as or safer than many of our other current treatments. Frankly, because of the wide range of research showing that it is safe and effective, it is almost inexcusable that it is not in wide use.

There is a paucity of effective treatments for bipolar I depression. For bipolar II/NOS, it is far worse. With this scarcity of effective treatments, it is imperative that we employ any and all medications that may help. Too many patients fail every medication or fail to reach full remission to ignore HDT. Yet despite all this, HDT is almost universally ignored.

Who Is in Charge: Are We Mice, or Are We Specialists?

The suffering that bipolar patients and their families undergo is immeasurable. The risk of suicide is ever present. The social risks of untreated or undertreated bipolar disorders are tremendous. Our patients suffer frequent job loss, prolonged unemployment, disability, divorce, family strife, violence, estrangement from family, incarceration, academic failure, substance abuse, substance dependence, bankruptcy, loss of friends, low self-esteem, repeated hospitalizations, misdiagnosis, and a multitude of other potential bad outcomes that are directly and indirectly related to the bipolar disorders. They drop out of psychiatric care due to frustration, loss of insurance, or, as is more common these days, being underinsured. Any one of these bad social outcomes can create an avalanche of other bad social outcomes. It is underappreciated that friends and family have limits as to what they can or will tolerate before they withdraw support, either in part or in whole, from an individual suffering from an unstable bipolar disorder. We have all watched the pain and suffering of our patients and their families as they drop down the socioeconomic ladder. Most of these patients could get well if they got the right treatments. The medical risks of untreated and undertreated bipolar disorders are many: weight gain, bad diet, obesity, diabetes, obstructive sleep apnea, smoking, poor care of existing medical problems, sexually transmitted diseases from hypersexuality, and the lack of physical activity that leads to osteoporosis, heart disease, and innumerable other bad medical outcomes that kill more people than suicide does.

The use of HDT is actively discouraged by a minority of endocrinologists based on the myth that HDT is equivalent to hyperthyroidism and the lack of understanding of the severe risks posed by the bipolar disorders. If you employ HDT, be prepared for pushback from other doctors, at least until HDT treatment is better understood. Doctors, NPs, PAs, pharmacists, patients' families, and even many psychiatrists who are not familiar with the research reviewed in this book will object to the use of HDT, equating low TSH and the high circulating level of T3 to hyperthyroidism.

To be frank, most nonpsychiatric physicians have little or no appreciation of the suffering that patients with a bipolar disorder endure. They lack a clear understanding of the social risks or the medical risks involved and thus are unable to develop an adequate risk-benefit analysis. Nonpsychiatric physicians rarely understand the risks or benefits of alternative psychiatric medications. This creates a dangerous situation as is evidenced by endocrinologists, internists, and other physicians who will routinely and without consulting the prescribing psychiatrist discontinue HDT without any consideration of the consequences when HDT is used to treat bipolar disorder. This is ironic in view of the fact that they promote the use of HDT to prevent thyroid cancer. The morbidity and mortality of the bipolar disorders outstrips the morbidity and mortality of thyroid cancer after the initial surgery has been performed.

It is imperative that psychiatrists (and psychiatric NPs) be in charge of treating bipolar disorders. Only psychiatrists are in the unique position to understand the risk and benefits of HDT. Only psychiatrists are in the position to know the risks of bipolar disorders. Only psychiatrists are in the position to know the risks of alternative medications.

The point is that psychiatrists should be in charge of treating bipolar patients. We should not tolerate interference from nonpsychiatrists. Simply put, nonpsychiatrists lack the requisite knowledge of the risks of bipolar or its treatments. We must keep in mind that <u>we are specialists!</u> Moreover, we are the only specialists who are equipped to treat these deadly illnesses we call bipolar disorders. For the sake of our patients, we must not cede treatment decisions to nonpsychiatrists. We must not allow ourselves to be steamrolled by physicians who are largely ignorant of the profound seriousness of the bipolar disorders and who are ignorant about the safety of HDT. Even if HDT carried the same risks as hyperthyroidism, there are many cases in which the risk-benefit analysis would still favor HDT! It is fine for other specialists to give their opinions about what they believe are the risks of a treatment, but they should not make treatment decisions.

HDT is not a panacea, nor is it risk-free. It doesn't work alone, and it doesn't work for all patients. All treatments come with risks. This includes HDT. Yet untreated bipolar disorders or even partially treated bipolar disorders carry far greater risks than any treatment does.

As shown in earlier chapters, HDT is as safe as or safer than any other treatment for bipolar disorder. It is efficacious and effective. Unlike so many other bipolar medications, it can help cognition and potentially could decrease the medical morbidity and mortality our patients.

Our patients are suffering. Some are dying. Our patients' families are suffering, and society at large is suffering from the effects of not treating or undertreating of bipolar disorders. Not having HDT as part of our armament to fight the bipolar disorders because of misguided criticism from other physicians or our own ignorance is a not only a failure in our role as psychiatrists but a failure of character.

Chapter 16: Summation

Medicine is a science of uncertainty and an art of probability.

–William Osler

Too many of our patients with bipolar disorders are dying prematurely. Patients with bipolar disorders are suffering, and their families are suffering. Too many of our patients are functionally and cognitively impaired. Such impairments are part of the bipolar illnesses, yet we compound the problems with our treatments. It is not enough to control symptoms; we should be helping patients return to full functioning. At the very least, we should avoid using medications that worsen functionality.

Strong Evidence for the Effectiveness

There are numerous small case series showing that HDT is beneficial for refractory bipolar depression. There is one large, long-term case series of 159 patients with refractory bipolar depression in which 84% of patients show significant improvement, with a full third going into long-term remission. What's more, the positive effects and remission were sustained for an average of almost two years, the study's observation time. Clinically, the benefits continued past the end of the study. The patients in this study and, in fact, most of the case series suffered from refractory bipolar depression and had exhausted evidence-based treatments. The patients in the case series were so ill that most would not be considered eligible for randomized, double-blind, placebo-controlled studies that pharmaceutical companies use to get FDA approval.

There is a randomized, double-blind, placebo-controlled study showing that HDT is efficacious. There is one failed randomized, double-blind, placebo-controlled study—failure being defined in the typical fashion: the treatment group showed improvement, but there was an inordinate placebo response, so the results failed to separate from placebo. No trials could be located that showed HDT did not help.

Proof of Proof

How many of the medications that we use to treat bipolar disorder actually show normalization of the neurophysiology of the brain associated with depressive symptoms? HDT does, and what's more, these improvements directly correlate with improvements of depression.

How Can We Not Use HDT?

Despite the fact that our evidence base for the treatment of bipolar disorders has been growing, most patients with bipolar depression quickly run through the available evidenced-based medications. Sure, ofttimes we can get patients less depressed. This is fine and good, but our goal is to make people well—"well" being defined as having little or no symptoms of the illness and returning to full functioning.

HDT is well tolerated, better than most bipolar medications.

Thyroid Hormone Treatment Is Not New to Psychiatry

Psychiatrists have been continuously using thyroid hormones for quite some time. Emil Kraepelin mentions using dried sheep thyroid to treat patients as far back as 1904. It is the single longest running treatment used by psychiatrists with the exception of psychotherapy.

Safety of HDT

How many of the medications we use to treat the bipolar disorders are associated with long-term morbidity and mortality (or, for that matter, short-term morbidity and mortality)? Worse, how many of the newer medications could have morbidity and mortality problems that we are not yet aware of?

Endocrinologists have been using HDT for quite some time to suppress the return of thyroid cancer. They have amassed more long-term safety data about HDT than is available for any psychiatric medication in use. The long-term safety data from psychiatry is equally without problems.

Contrast the Results of HDT and Antidepressants

Despite the fact that antidepressants are controversial, not efficacious, and of questionable value, they continued to be widely used. Contrast HDT with antidepressants: HDT does not cause mania, does not cause rapid cycling, does not cause suicide, does not kill sexual drive, does not cause erectile dysfunction, does not cause dizziness, does not make patients tired, does not cause weight gain, is not difficult to discontinue, and does not cause osteoporosis (unlike SSRIs, valproic acid, and carbamazepine). It is much less expensive than antidepressants that are still under patent and of equivalent cost to generic antidepressants. Most importantly, the response and remission rates in bipolar depression are far better with HDT than with antidepressants.

A Theory with Great Possibilities

The theory of how HDT works is fascinating. Having a medication that does not increase medical morbidity and mortality is helpful, but if the theory is correct, HDT could go much farther than that. How exciting would it be if we could not only prolong our patients' lives but improve the quality by decreasing the medical problems associated with bipolar disorders? HDT may actually do this. The HDT theory is that the high circulating levels of thyroid hormone increase the gradient of passive diffusion to reverse cellular hypothyroidism. It may not be a coincidence that the medical morbidity and mortality of the bipolar disorders are similar to the morbidity and mortality of hypothyroidism. Thus, HDT would correct cellular hypothyroidism. The jury is still out on this. The theory is certainly compelling and deserves further research.

What percentage of patients with bipolar disorders show improvement but are not well? If this theory is correct, many of these patients may never be well until we treat their cellular hypothyroidism.

Cognition

Although HDT has not been formally shown to improve cognition, it has been shown to lessen the cognitive dysfunction from ECT beyond just decreasing the number of treatments. The overwhelming clinical experience of working with many highly educated individuals and the fact that it displaced widespread use of donepezil shows that it can be quite beneficial. It can be successful to the point that other cognitive treatments are not necessary.

If HDT Were a New Drug

HDT is an orphaned medication. There are no patents on any of the thyroid hormones. If HDT were a new treatment owned by a pharmaceutical company, that company would be pouring a billion dollars into research and another three hundred million for marketing. There would be an army of drug reps knocking at our doors, eager to tell us all about HDT. As psychiatrists, we must not be content to be spoon-fed information by drug reps. We must be aware of and make special effort to be familiar with orphaned medications.

HDT Is Not Hyperthyroidism

Perhaps the biggest roadblock to the use of HDT is the mistaken belief that it is equivalent to hyperthyroidism. Nothing could be farther from the truth. If it were equivalent to hyperthyroidism, endocrinologists would not be using HDT to prevent the return of thyroid cancer. If HDT were equivalent to hyperthyroidism, we would expect the same medical morbidity and mortality we see with hyperthyroidism. Instead, with HDT we see no increase in morbidity and mortality. Hyperthyroidism is an autoimmune disease, and its morbidity and mortality seem to be related to the autoimmune components of the illness.

To be sure, too much thyroid hormone can cause thyrotoxicity whether the source is external or endogenous. This is minimized with HDT by a careful titration and simply dealt with by reducing the dose if thyrotoxic symptoms appear.

HDT Is Recommended in Major Treatment Guidelines

HDT has been recommended over the years in many bipolar treatment guidelines. The two latest and most important are the Texas Medication Algorithm Project *Procedure Manual for Bipolar Disorder* and the Canadian Network for Mood and Anxiety

Treatments and International Society for Bipolar Disorders collaborative update in 2013 of CANMAT guidelines for the management of patients with bipolar disorder.

It's Not a Panacea

Nothing in this book should imply that HDT works for every patient or that there are no risks. HDT is not a first-line medication. It doesn't work alone, and it must be combined with other bipolar treatments. Clinically, it's usually added after the first three or four medications are not enough to reach euthymia. No medicine works for all, and no medicine is wholly without risks. The book provides more than sufficient evidence to show that HDT should be utilized.

This book has pulled together and documented the relevant facts about HDT from the more-than-adequate evidence base but also the clinical wisdom amassed in thirty-plus years of using thyroid hormone.

The Question

Again, the question is not, why should we use high-dose thyroid? The question is, why are we not using high-dose thyroid?

Appendix

Abbreviations

ECT = Electroconvulsive therapy

EEG = electroencephalogram

FDG-PET = [F-18] fluorodeoxyglucose, positron emission tomographic

HDT = high-dose thyroid

HR = hazard ratio

Li = lithium

MDQ = Mood Disorder Questionnaire

OR = odds ratio

rT3 = Reverse T3

SSRI = selective serotonin reuptake inhibitors

TSHr = TSH receptor antibodies

Patient information handout:

Thyroid Hormone Information for the Treatment of the Bipolar Disorders

High-dose thyroid = HDT

A few thoughts about risks: Most likely, the single biggest risk to your health is uncontrolled bipolar disorder. The second-biggest risk to your health is partially controlled bipolar disorder. If you need HDT and it works, it is far safer to continue it than not to take it. When in doubt, ask me. Other doctors who are not familiar with the scientific literature will disagree.

Thyroid hormones come in two types: **T4, called levothyroxine**, and **T3, called liothyronine**. (Note that 25 mcg of T3 is equal to about 100 mcg of T4). T3 is preferred for the treatment of the bipolar disorders and depression because it is much easier and quicker to get to therapeutic doses. T3 is much less affected by eating, and the dose can be increased as quickly as every week. With T4, it is difficult to increase the dose more than every four to five weeks. There are other theoretical reasons to prefer T3.

When can I expect help: T3 usually works somewhere between two and five pills (25 mcg each), sometimes less; sometimes more. This can be as quick as two to five weeks, depending on how often you can come in.

Side effects: The bottom line is that side effects from HDT are mild, for the most part, and easily dealt with. It is unusual that side effects cause the need to stop thyroid hormone. The usual side effects that we watch for are the following:

1. If you are feeling hot all the time, your thyroid dose may be too high. This sometimes comes in the form of hot flashes. (If you already have hot flashes, we would be looking for an increase in hot flashes.) Hot flashes that exclusively happen early in the morning (usually between 1:00 a.m. and 6:00 a.m.) can be handled by moving some of the thyroid dose to evening.

2. We follow your heart rate to make sure it stays below one hundred (when relaxed and comfortable). When you exercise, we expect that your heart rate will go above 100 *as it does naturally.*
3. While thyroid hormone can be very helpful for anxiety, too much can increase anxiety. It is important to tell me doctor right away if after starting or increasing your thyroid dose, your anxiety worsens.
4. A little bit of tremor is OK. You are the one who decides what is too much. If you experience tremor when you crouch or step on the brakes of your car, reduce your dose by one-half pill and call me.
5. Extremely rare side effect: If when first starting thyroid, you get severe joint and muscle pain, usually in the hands and feet, stop the thyroid. You won't have to guess at this. It happens in about one out of 300 patients.
6. Rare side effect: If we get up to higher doses, some patients can experience bone, joint, or muscle pain. This is usually mild and is often misattributed to other causes. Please report any type of muscular or joint pain that is not obviously from an injury or a hard workout.
7. Rare side effect: Heart arrhythmias and atrial fibrillation. Research shows that long-term HDT does not cause atrial fibrillation. I'm not sure this is correct, but since atrial fibrillation happens to people who are not on HDT, it is hard to judge. This is one of the reasons we keep the resting heart rate below 100. If atrial fibrillation does develop, it is easily handled by a dose reduction or other methods. Case reports indicate that once atrial fibrillation has stopped, HDT can be carefully reintroduced without the redevelopment of atrial fibrillation.

There are a number of other side effects that overlap depressive symptoms, so if there are any other changes in your body or mood (for the worse) it is important that you let me know.

Effects on weight: Only a small number of patients will lose a lot of weight. Many others can experience increased appetite without weight gain. Overall, except for the few who lose weight, thyroid hormone is weight-neutral.

Safety: The scientific literature shows that HDT is as safe as or safer than most of the alternative medicines we could use. If it works, it is far safer to take it than not to take it.

Other doctors: The use of HDT is highly specialized. Despite the fact HDT is recommended in multiple treatment guidelines, most doctors are not aware of the research showing that HDT is as safe as or safer than other medicines used to treat bipolar disorders. They may mistakenly equate HDT with causing hyperthyroidism. It does not cause hyperthyroidism. The scientific literature shows that external thyroid is not associated with osteoporosis, heart problems, or early death. Most doctors are not aware of this and may tell you that you need to decrease your dose or stop it all together. If this happens, insist that they talk to me first. If indeed you are having side effects from too much thyroid, then a small decrease of your thyroid dose is in order. However, keep in mind that what you believe is a side effect could be caused by another medication or may even be a feature of your illness. You should talk to me before decreasing the dose. If you are forced to decrease your dose, please don't decrease it more than 12.5 to 25 mcg, and talk to me as soon as it is practical.

How does HDT help my symptoms? We think that people with a bipolar disorders and depressions have difficulties getting thyroid hormone from their blood into the cells of your body (where thyroid hormone works). This results in low levels of thyroid hormones inside your cells even if tests show "normal levels" in your blood. In other words, even if your tests show normal blood levels, thyroid hormone levels inside cells can be low. The extra thyroid hormone helps "push" enough thyroid hormone into your cells.

Should I get thyroid hormone blood levels? No, in this circumstance blood levels of thyroid hormone to not predict thyroid levels inside cells. We monitor your levels the old-fashioned way. If you're bipolar and you are well, your levels are good. If you have symptoms of too much thyroid hormone (usually mild) then you are on too much.

Does HDT help everyone? Sorry, no. No medication helps everyone.

Who recommends the use of HDT? HDT is recommended in two major treatment guidelines for the treatment of bipolar depression. HDT is also used by endocrinologists to prevent the return of thyroid cancer.

Model letter to other physicians involved in the treatment of your patient:

The following letter can be used as is or modified in any way you wish. The main purposes of the letter are to start educating other physicians about the use of HDT and to discourage them from actions that will endanger patients—that is, abruptly stopping HDT.

HIGH-DOSE THYROID

RE:

DOB:

Dear Dr.[name],

I am writing to let you know that I am recommending the use of high-dose thyroid (HDT) for our common patient. [Name of patient] is suffering a serious bipolar disorder. The patient has tried and failed a number of other medications.

HDT is highly effective for treating bipolar disorders. Keep in mind that the morbidity and mortality of bipolar disorders are often underappreciated. On average, patients with bipolar disorder die 20 years early. Surprisingly, suicide accounts for about one-quarter of premature deaths. Most mortality from bipolar disorder comes from cardiovascular complications. Also underappreciated are the significant risks from many of the bipolar medications. For most patients, the risk-benefit analysis favors a trial of HDT. Please keep in mind that endocrinologists routinely use HDT to prevent the return of thyroid cancer. The morbidity and mortality of nontreated or undertreated bipolar disorders are higher than those of thyroid cancers after the initial thyroid ablation.

Historically, the use of HDT is recommended by four of the most well-respected bipolar treatment guidelines. Its efficacy is well established. The use of HDT often results in a suppressed TSH and, usually but not always, elevation of T4 and T3. If T3 is used, the TSH and T4 levels will likely be suppressed and T3 levels will likely be elevated. If T4 is used, expect low TSH with elevated T4 and T3 levels. Most importantly, HDT is not hyperthyroidism and cannot cause hyperthyroidism. By definition, hyperthyroidism is a set of symptoms consistent with thyrotoxicity, with an overproduction of endogenous thyroid hormone. This is a very important distinction for the following reasons:

1) HDT is remarkably well tolerated in patients with affective illnesses.
2) It turns out that most, if not all, sequelae of hyperthyroidism come from an autoimmune process. These include osteoporosis and the cardiovascular risks. The autoimmune problems persist even after thyroid ablation.
3) HDT has been extensively tested in thyroid cancer, where it suppresses the return of thyroid cancer. A careful review of the research shows that external HDT does not cause bone loss, nor does it increase mortality or morbidity.
4) Many of the other alternative psychiatric medications do carry a risk for osteoporosis and have the potential to increase mortality or morbidity. In addition, HDT carries no fall risk, while most psychiatric medications do.

How does HDT work? Neuroimaging of the bipolar disorders has shown that HDT decreases brain metabolism in areas that are connected to depression. How? Research has established that patients with a bipolar disorder have low ATP levels secondary to mitochondrial dysfunction. Getting thyroid hormones across cell membranes is an energy-intensive process that requires ATP. This makes it difficult to get T4 and T3 across cell membranes and creates cellular hypothyroidism. The high blood levels of thyroid drive more thyroid hormone into cells, compensating for the lack of active transport. The only exception to the cellular hypothyroidism is the pituitary, where both T3 and T4 enter by passive means. The practical results, prior to the HDT treatment, are that patients suffering from affective disorders can have normal thyroid blood levels because the pituitary "sees" normal blood levels despite the fact of low cellular thyroid levels. When high-dose thyroid is given, the pituitary "sees" the high levels (thus the low TSH), but the rest of the body gets the thyroid it needs. Research has shown that HDT can be very effective at treating bipolar disorders and is safe.

In sum, the use of high-dose thyroid is certainly less risky than use of most of the alternative psychiatric medications. It usually does not cause thyrotoxicity, either. Because so many thyrotoxic symptoms resemble symptoms of bipolar disorders (for example, palpitations, anxiety, or panic attacks) or could be side effects of other psychiatric medications (for example, tremor or hair loss), please refer the patient back to me if you find possible thyrotoxic symptoms. The worst thing you can do is to abruptly stop high-dose thyroid. Abruptly stopping high-dose thyroid has been shown to cause permanent damage to the heart and possibly to other organs. Abruptly stopping the thyroid hormone puts the patient at profound risk for relapse with a concomitant risk of suicide. If the dose must be decreased, please decrease it only by 12.5 mcg to 25 mcg. If T4 is being used, reduce it by 50 mcg to 100 mcg but no further. I will handle further dosage decreases if they are needed.

I do understand that this is a paradigm shift in our thinking about thyroid hormones and runs counter to what we were all taught. Most of us were taught in medical school that in by 10 years, half of what we thought was true will be eclipsed by further research. This is one of those instances. Psychiatrists have been hard at work developing a risks/benefit/safety analysis of HDT. The use of HDT is recommended by the most respected and the most current treatment guidelines developed by Canadian government and the International Bipolar Disorder Society.

Atrial fibrillation: Atrial fibrillation is surprisingly rare with HDT and usually easily handled. If you find a patient on HDT that as developed atrial fibrillation, keep in mind that it may not necessarily be caused by the HDT—or at least the HDT alone. Keep in mind that for some patients, the risk of stopping the HDT far outweighs the risk of atrial fibrillation. Often the simple steps of starting a beta blocker and/or stopping all caffeine will stop atrial fibrillation. Keep in mind that there's never been a documented case of ventricular fibrillation with HDT and that ventricular fibrillation is extremely rare even in full-blown hyperthyroidism.

If you have any concerns about HDT and/or want to decrease the dose of thyroid, please contact me so we can develop a risk-benefit analysis together.

If you wish, I can provide references for the safety and efficacy of HDT on request. Send the request to [contact information of your practice].

Sincerely,

References

Abonowara, A., Quraishi, A., Sapp, J.L., Alqambar, M.H., Saric, A., O'Connell, C.M., Rajaraman, M.M., Hart, R.D., Imran, S.A., 2012. Prevalence of atrial fibrillation in patients taking TSH suppression therapy for management of thyroid cancer. Clinical & Investigative Medicine 35, E152-E156.

Akslen, L.A., Haldorsen, T., Thoresen, S.Ø., Glattre, E., 1991. Survival and causes of death in thyroid cancer: a population-based study of 2479 cases from Norway. Cancer Res. 51, 1234-1241.

Bahn, R.S., Burch, H.B., Cooper, D.S., Garber, J.R., Greenlee, M.C., Klein, I., Laurberg, P., McDougall, I.R., Montori, V.M., Rivkees, S.A., 2011. Hyperthyroidism and other causes of thyrotoxicosis: management guidelines of the American Thyroid Association and American Association of Clinical Endocrinologists. Thyroid 21, 593-646.

Bailey, B., McGuigan, M., 2000. Lithium poisoning from a poison control center perspective. Therapeutic drug monitoring 22, 650-655.

Bauer, M., Adli, M., Bschor, T., Heinz, A., Rasgon, N., Frye, M., Grunze, H., Kupka, R., Whybrow, P., 2003. Clinical applications of levothyroxine in refractory mood disorders. Clin Appl Bipolar Disord 2, 49-56.

Bauer, M., Baur, H., Berghöfer, A., Ströhle, A., Hellweg, R., Müller-Oerlinghausen, B., Baumgartner, A., 2002. Effects of supraphysiological thyroxine administration in healthy controls and patients with depressive disorders. J. Affect. Disord. 68, 285-294.

Bauer, M., Berman, S., Stamm, T., Plotkin, M., Adli, M., Pilhatsch, M., London, E., Hellemann, G., Whybrow, P., Schlagenhauf, F., 2015. Levothyroxine effects on depressive symptoms and limbic glucose metabolism in bipolar disorder: a randomized, placebo-controlled positron emission tomography study. Mol. Psychiatry.

Bauer, M., Fairbanks, L., Berghöfer, A., Hierholzer, J., Bschor, T., Baethge, C., Rasgon, N., Sasse, J., Whybrow, P.C., 2004. Bone mineral density during maintenance treatment with supraphysiological doses of levothyroxine in affective disorders: a longitudinal study. J. Affect. Disord. 83, 183-190.

Bauer, M., London, E., Rasgon, N., Berman, S., Frye, M., Altshuler, L., Mandelkern, M., Bramen, J., Voytek, B., Woods, R., 2005. Supraphysiological doses of levothyroxine alter regional cerebral metabolism and improve mood in bipolar depression. Mol. Psychiatry 10, 456-469.

Bauer, M., Whybrow, P.C., 2001. Thyroid hormone, neural tissue and mood modulation. World J. Biol. Psychiatry 2, 59-69.

Bauer, M.S., Whybrow, P.C., 1990. Rapid cycling bipolar affective disorder: II. Treatment of refractory rapid cycling with high-dose levothyroxine: A preliminary study. Arch. Gen. Psychiatry 47, 435.

Belaya, Z.E., Melnichenko, G.A., Rozhinskaya, L.Y., Fadeev, V.V., Alekseeva, T.M., Dorofeeva, O.K., Sasonova, N.I., Kolesnikova, G.S., 2007. Subclinical hyperthyroidism of variable etiology and its influence on bone in postmenopausal women. HORMONES-ATHENS- 6, 62.

Benvenga, S., 2013. When thyroid hormone replacement is ineffective? Current Opinion in Endocrinology, Diabetes and Obesity 20, 467-477.

Berken, G.H., Weinstein, D.O., Stern, W.C., 1984. Weight gain: a side-effect of tricyclic antidepressants. Journal of affective disorders 7, 133-138.

Biondi, B., 2012. Mechanisms in endocrinology: heart failure and thyroid dysfunction. European Journal of Endocrinology 167, 609-618.

Biondi, B., Kahaly, G.J., 2010. Cardiovascular involvement in patients with different causes of hyperthyroidism. Nature Reviews Endocrinology 6, 431-443.

Bodén, R., Lundgren, M., Brandt, L., Reutfors, J., Andersen, M., Kieler, H., 2012. Risks of adverse pregnancy and birth outcomes in women treated or not treated with mood stabilisers for bipolar disorder: population based cohort study. bmj 345, e7085.

Boeker, H., Seidl, A., Schopper, C., 2011. Neurotoxicity related to combined treatment with lithium, antidepressants and atypical antipsychotics. Schweizer Archiv Fur Neurologie Und Psychiatrie 162, 72-76.

Bruyère, O., Reginster, J.-Y., 2015. Osteoporosis in patients taking selective serotonin reuptake inhibitors: a focus on fracture outcome. Endocrine 48, 65-68.

Bryant, A.E., Dreifuss, F.E., 1996. Valproic acid hepatic fatalities. III. US experience since 1986. Neurology 46, 465-469.

Celi, F.S., Zemskova, M., Linderman, J.D., Smith, S., Drinkard, B., Sachdev, V., Skarulis, M.C., Kozlosky, M., Csako, G., Costello, R., 2011. Metabolic effects of liothyronine therapy in hypothyroidism: a randomized, double-blind, crossover trial of liothyronine versus levothyroxine. The Journal of Clinical Endocrinology & Metabolism 96, 3466-3474.

Chakrabarti, S., 2011. Thyroid functions and bipolar affective disorder. J. Thyroid Res. 2011.

Chang, C.M., Wu, E.C.H., Chen, C.Y., Wu, K.Y., Liang, H.Y., Chau, Y.L., Wu, C.S., Lin, K.M., Tsai, H.J., 2013. Psychotropic drugs and risk of motor vehicle accidents: a population-based case-control study. British journal of clinical pharmacology 75, 1125-1133.

Chen, C.-H., Chen, J.-F., Yang, B.-Y., Liu, R.-T., Tung, S.-C., Chien, W.-Y., Lu, Y.-C., Kuo, M.-C., Hsieh, C.-J., Wang, P.-W., 2004. Bone mineral density in women receiving thyroxine suppressive therapy for differentiated thyroid carcinoma. Journal of the Formosan Medical Association= Taiwan yi zhi 103, 442-447.

Cheng, Y.X., Chong, C.P., 2013. A case report of a bipolar disorder patient with severe lithium poisoning possibly induced by interaction between risperidone, telmisartan, fluvoxamine and lithium. Journal of Applied Pharmaceutical Science Vol 3, S79-S82.

Cole, D.P., Thase, M.E., Mallinger, A.G., Soares, J.C., Luther, J.F., Kupfer, D.J., Frank, E., 2002. Slower treatment response in bipolar depression predicted by lower pretreatment thyroid function. Am. J. Psychiatry 159, 116-121.

Cooper, D.S., Doherty, G.M., Haugen, B.R., Kloos, R.T., Lee, S.L., Mandel, S.J., Mazzaferri, E.L., McIver, B., Pacini, F., Schlumberger, M., 2009. Revised american thyroid association management guidelines for patients with thyroid nodules and differentiated thyroid cancer: the american thyroid association (ATA) guidelines taskforce on thyroid nodules and differentiated thyroid cancer. Thyroid 19, 1167-1214.

Corn, T., Checkley, S., 1983. A case of recurrent mania with recurrent hyperthyroidism. Br. J. Psychiatry 142, 74-76.

Crismon, M.L., Argo, T.R., Bendele, S.D., Suppes, T., 2007. Texas Medication Algorithm Project Procdural Manual, Bipolar Disorder Algorithms. Texas Department of State Health Services.

De-yuan, H., 2009. serotonin syndrome: history and risk. Fundamental & Clinical Pharmacology.

De Groot, L., Abalovich, M., Alexander, E.K., Amino, N., Barbour, L., Cobin, R.H., Eastman, C.J., Lazarus, J.H., Luton, D., Mandel, S.J., 2012. Management of thyroid dysfunction during pregnancy and postpartum: an Endocrine Society clinical practice guideline. The Journal of Clinical Endocrinology & Metabolism 97, 2543-2565.

Diem, S.J., Blackwell, T.L., Stone, K.L., Yaffe, K., Haney, E.M., Bliziotes, M.M., Ensrud, K.E., 2007. Use of antidepressants and rates of hip bone loss in older women: the study of osteoporotic fractures. Arch. Intern. Med. 167, 1240-1245.

Dietrich, J., Brisseau, K., Boehm, B., 2008. [Absorption, transport and bioavailability of iodothyronines]. Deutsche medizinische Wochenschrift (1946) 133, 1644-1648.

Drvota, V., Janson, A., Norman, C., Sylven, C., Haggblad, J., Bronnegard, M., Marcus, C., 1995. Evidence for the presence of functional thyrotropin receptor in cardiac muscle. Biochem. Biophys. Res. Commun. 211, 426-431.

Duval, F., Mokrani, M.-C., Lopera, F.G., Diep, T.S., Rabia, H., Fattah, S., 2010. Thyroid axis activity and suicidal behavior in depressed patients. Psychoneuroendocrinology 35, 1045-1054.

Eftekhari, M., Asadollahi, A., Beiki, D., Izadyar, S., Gholamrezanezhad, A., Assadi, M., Fard-Esfahani, A., Fallahi, B., Takavar, A., Saghari, M., 2008. The long term effect of levothyroxine on bone mineral density in patients with well differentiated thyroid carcinoma after treatment. Hell. J. Nucl. Med. 11, 160-163.

Escobar-Morreale, H.F., Obregón, M.J., Del Rey, F.E., De Escobar, G.M., 1995. Replacement therapy for hypothyroidism with thyroxine alone does not ensure euthyroidism in all tissues, as studied in thyroidectomized rats. Journal of Clinical Investigation 96, 2828.

Everts, M.E., de JONG, M., Lim, C.-F., Docter, R., Krenning, E.P., Visser, T.J., Hennemann, G., 1996. Different regulation of thyroid hormone transport in liver and pituitary: its possible role in the maintenance of low T3 production during nonthyroidal illness and fasting in man. Thyroid 6, 359-368.

Fadel, B.M., Ellahham, S., Lindsay, J., Ringel, M.D., Wartofsky, L., Burman, K.D., 2000. Hyperthyroid heart disease. Clin. Cardiol. 23, 402-408.

Fagiolini, A., Frank, E., Houck, P.R., Mallinger, A.G., Swartz, H.A., Buysse, D.J., Ombao, H., Kupfer, D.J., 2002. Prevalence of obesity and weight change during treatment in patients with bipolar I disorder. Journal of Clinical Psychiatry 63, 528-533.

Fazio, S., Palmieri, E.A., Lombardi, G., Biondi, B., 2004. Effects of thyroid hormone on the cardiovascular system. Recent Prog. Horm. Res. 59, 31-50.

Frye, M.A., Denicoff, K.D., Bryan, A.L., Smith-Jackson, E.E., Ali, S.O., Luckenbaugh, D., Leverich, G.S., Post, R.M., 1999. Association between lower serum free T4 and greater mood instability and depression in lithium-maintained bipolar patients. American Journal of Psychiatry.

Frye, M.A., Ha, K., Kanba, S., Kato, T., Özerdem, A., Vázquez, G., Vieta, E., 2011. International consensus group on depression prevention in bipolar disorder. The Journal of clinical psychiatry 72, 1295.

Garber, J.R., Cobin, R.H., Gharib, H., Hennessey, J.V., Klein, I., Mechanick, J.I., Pessah-Pollack, R., Singer, P.A., Woeber, K.A., 2012. Clinical practice guidelines for hypothyroidism in adults: cosponsored by the American Association of Clinical Endocrinologists and the American Thyroid Association. Endocrine Practice 18, 988-1028.

Gershengorn, M.C., Neumann, S., 2012. Update in TSH Receptor Agonists and Antagonists. The Journal of Clinical Endocrinology & Metabolism 97, 4287-4292.

Gibson, J.E., Hubbard, R.B., Smith, C.J., Tata, L.J., Britton, J.R., Fogarty, A.W., 2009. Use of self-controlled analytical techniques to assess the association between use of prescription medications and the risk of motor vehicle crashes. American journal of epidemiology, kwn364.

Go, A.S., Hylek, E.M., Phillips, K.A., Chang, Y., Henault, L.E., Selby, J.V., Singer, D.E., 2001. Prevalence of diagnosed atrial fibrillation in adults: national implications for rhythm management and stroke prevention: the AnTicoagulation and Risk Factors in Atrial Fibrillation (ATRIA) Study. JAMA 285, 2370-2375.

Green, M.F., 2006. Cognitive impairment and functional outcome in schizophrenia and bipolar disorder. The Journal of clinical psychiatry 67, 3-8.

Gyulai, L., Bauer, M., Garcia-Espana, F., Hierholzer, J., Baumgartner, A., Berghöfer, A., Whybrow, P.C., 2001. Bone mineral density in pre-and post-menopausal women with affective disorder treated with long-term L-thyroxine augmentation. J. Affect. Disord. 66, 185-191.

Gyulai, L., Jaggi, J., Bauer, M.S., Younkin, S., Rubin, L., Attie, M., Whybrow, P.C., 1997. Bone mineral density and L-thyroxine treatment in rapidly cycling bipolar disorder. Biol. Psychiatry 41, 503-506.

Halbreich, U., Rojansky, N., Palter, S., Hreshchyshyn, M., Kreeger, J., Bakhai, Y., Rosan, R., 1995. Decreased bone mineral density in medicated psychiatric patients. Psychosomatic Medicine 57, 485-491.

Haugen, B.R., Alexander, E.K., Bible, K.C., Doherty, G.M., Mandel, S.J., Nikiforov, Y.E., Pacini, F., Randolph, G.W., Sawka, A.M., Schlumberger, M., 2016. 2015 American Thyroid Association management guidelines for adult patients with thyroid nodules and differentiated thyroid cancer: the American Thyroid Association guidelines task force on thyroid nodules and differentiated thyroid cancer. Thyroid 26, 1-133.

Heemstra, K., Hamdy, N., Romijn, J., Smit, J., 2006. The effects of thyrotropin-suppressive therapy on bone metabolism in patients with well-differentiated thyroid carcinoma. Thyroid 16, 583-591.

Heeringa, J., van der Kuip, D.A., Hofman, A., Kors, J.A., van Herpen, G., Stricker, B.H.C., Stijnen, T., Lip, G.Y., Witteman, J.C., 2006. Prevalence, incidence and lifetime risk of atrial fibrillation: the Rotterdam study. European heart journal 27, 949-953.

Hennemann, G., Docter, R., Friesema, E.C., de Jong, M., Krenning, E.P., Visser, T.J., 2001. Plasma membrane transport of thyroid hormones and its role in thyroid hormone metabolism and bioavailability. Endocrine reviews 22, 451-476.

Hesselink, E.N.K., Hesselink, M.S.K., de Bock, G.H., Gansevoort, R.T., Bakker, S.J., Vredeveld, E.J., van der Horst-Schrivers, A.N., van der Horst, I.C., Kamphuisen, P.W., Plukker, J.T., 2013. Long-term cardiovascular mortality in patients with differentiated thyroid carcinoma: an observational study. J. Clin. Oncol., JCO. 2013.2049. 1043.

Higashiguchi, M., Onoda, T., Turin, T.C., Sakata, K., 2009. Calcium intake and associated factors in a general Japanese population: baseline data of NIPPON DATA80/90 and the National Nutrition Survey. Journal of epidemiology/Japan Epidemiological Association 20, S549-556.

Hirschfeld, R., 2010. Guideline watch: Practice guideline for the treatment of patients with bipolar disorder, APA Practice Guidelines. Am Psychiatric Assoc.

Hirschfeld, R.M., Cass, A.R., Holt, D.C., Carlson, C.A., 2005. Screening for bipolar disorder in patients treated for depression in a family medicine clinic. The Journal of the American board of family practice 18, 233-239.

Holtorf, K., 2014. Thyroid Hormone Transport into Cellular Tissue. Journal of Restorative Medicine 3, 53-68.

Hubert, H.B., Feinleib, M., McNamara, P.M., Castelli, W.P., 1983. Obesity as an independent risk factor for cardiovascular disease: a 26-year follow-up of participants in the Framingham Heart Study. Circulation 67, 968-977.

Jacobsen, F., Comas-Díaz, L., 1999. Donepezil for psychotropic-induced memory loss. The Journal of clinical psychiatry 60, 698.

Jodar, E., Lopez, M.B., Garcia, L., Rigopoulou, D., Martinez, G., Hawkins, F., 1998. Bone changes in pre-and postmenopausal women with thyroid cancer on levothyroxine therapy: evolution of axial and appendicular bone mass. Osteoporos. Int. 8, 311-316.

Jonklaas, J., Sarlis, N.J., Litofsky, D., Ain, K.B., Bigos, S.T., Brierley, J.D., Cooper, D.S., Haugen, B.R., Ladenson, P.W., Magner, J., 2006. Outcomes of patients with differentiated thyroid carcinoma following initial therapy. Thyroid 16, 1229-1242.

Jou, S.-H., Chiu, N.-Y., Liu, C.-S., 2009. Mitochondrial dysfunction and psychiatric disorders. Chang Gung Med. J. 32, 370-379.

Kalra, S., Khandelwal, S.K., 2011. Why are our hypothyroid patients unhappy? Is tissue hypothyroidism the answer? Indian J. Endocrinol. Metab. 15, S95.

Keaepelin, E., 1902. Clinical Psychiatry A Textbook for Students and Physicians abstracted and Adapted from the Six German Edition of Kraepelin's "Lehrubch Der Psychiatrie". THE MACMILLAN COMPANY New York/LONDON: MACMILLAN& CO., Ltd.

Kelly, T., 2008. Is donepezil useful for improving cognitive dysfunction in bipolar disorder? J. Affect. Disord. 107, 237-240.

Kelly, T., 2014. A favorable risk-benefit analysis of High dose thyroid for treatment of bipolar Disorders with regard to osteoporosis. J. Affect. Disord.

Kelly, T., 2015. An examination of myth: A favorable cardiovascular risk-benefit analysis of high-dose thyroid for affective disorders. J. Affect. Disord. 177, 49-58.

Kelly, T., 2016. Diagnostic interviews: work smarter not harder. The psychiatric newsletter, editor Nassir Ghaemi, 7-8.

Kelly, T., Douglas, L., Denmark, L., Brasuell, G., Lieberman, D.Z., 2013. The high prevalence of obstructive sleep apnea among patients with bipolar disorders. J. Affect. Disord. 151, 54-58.

Kelly, T., Lieberman, D.Z., 2009. The use of triiodothyronine as an augmentation agent in treatment-resistant bipolar II and bipolar disorder NOS. Journal of affective disorders 116, 222-226.

Kelly, T., Lieberman, D.Z., 2017. The Utility of Low-Dose Aripiprazole for the Treatment of Bipolar II and Bipolar NOS Depression. J. Clin. Psychopharmacol. 37, 99-101.

Klein, I., Danzi, S., 2007. Thyroid disease and the heart. Circulation 116, 1725-1735.

Köhrle, J., 2007. Thyroid hormone transporters in health and disease: advances in thyroid hormone deiodination. Best Practice & Research Clinical Endocrinology & Metabolism 21, 173-191.

Kono, S., Sunagawa, Y., Higa, H., Sunagawa, H., 1990. Age of menopause in Japanese women: trends and recent changes. Maturitas 12, 43-49.

Kraepelin, E., 1899. Lehrubuch Der Psyciatrie, Sixth Edition.

Krhin, B., Besic, N., 2012. Effectiveness of L-thyroxine treatment on TSH suppression during pregnancy in patients with a history of thyroid carcinoma after total thyroidectomy and radioiodine ablation. Radiology and oncology 46, 160-165.

Kung, A., Yeung, S., 1996. Prevention of bone loss induced by thyroxine suppressive therapy in postmenopausal women: the effect of calcium and calcitonin. The Journal of Clinical Endocrinology & Metabolism 81, 1232-1236.

Kung, A.W., Lorentz, T., Tam, S.C., 1993. Thyroxine suppressive therapy decreases bone mineral density in post-menopausal women. Clinical endocrinology 39, 535-540.

Kung, A.W., Ng, F., 1994. A rat model of thyroid hormone-induced bone loss: effect of antiresorptive agents on regional bone density and osteocalcin gene expression. Thyroid 4, 93-98.

Laurberg, P., Wallin, G., Tallstedt, L., Abraham-Nordling, M., Lundell, G., Tørring, O., 2008. TSH-receptor autoimmunity in Graves' disease after therapy with anti-thyroid drugs, surgery, or radioiodine: a 5-year prospective randomized study. European Journal of Endocrinology 158, 69-75.

Laursen, T.M., 2011. Life expectancy among persons with schizophrenia or bipolar affective disorder. Schizophrenia research 131, 101-104.

Leboyer, M., Soreca, I., Scott, J., Frye, M., Henry, C., Tamouza, R., Kupfer, D.J., 2012. Can bipolar disorder be viewed as a multi-system inflammatory disease? J. Affect. Disord. 141, 1-10.

Lee, S., Chow, C.C., Wing, Y., Leung, C., Chiu, H., Chen, C., 1991. Mania secondary to thyrotoxicosis. Br. J. Psychiatry 159, 712-713.

Links, T., Van Tol, K., Jager, P., Plukker, J.T.M., Piers, D., Boezen, H., Dullaart, R., de Vries, E., Sluiter, W., 2005. Life expectancy in differentiated thyroid cancer: a novel approach to survival analysis. Endocr. Relat. Cancer 12, 273-280.

Lloyd-Jones, D.M., Wang, T.J., Leip, E.P., Larson, M.G., Levy, D., Vasan, R.S., D'Agostino, R.B., Massaro, J.M., Beiser, A., Wolf, P.A., 2004. Lifetime risk for development of atrial fibrillation. Circulation 110, 1042-1046.

Magalhaes, P., Kapczinski, F., Nierenberg, A., Deckersbach, T., Weisinger, D., Dodd, S., Berk, M., 2012. Illness burden and medical comorbidity in the Systematic Treatment Enhancement Program for Bipolar Disorder. Acta psychiatrica scandinavica 125, 303-308.

Mandel, S.J.L., P. Reed; Davis, Terry F, 2011. Thyrotoxicosis, In: Kronenberg, H.M.L., P. Reed;Melmed, Shlomo;Polonsky, Kenneth S;Williams, Robert H (Ed.), Williams Textbook of Endocrinology. 12th ed. Elsevier/Saunders, Philadelphia, pp. 362-405.

Manji, H., Kato, T., Di Prospero, N.A., Ness, S., Beal, M.F., Krams, M., Chen, G., 2012. Impaired mitochondrial function in psychiatric disorders. Nature Reviews Neuroscience 13, 293-307.

Mansourian, A.R., 2010. A review on hyperthyroidism: thyrotoxicosis under surveillance. Pakistan Journal of Biological Sciences 13, 1066.

Meaney, A.M., Smith, S., Howes, O., O'brien, M., Murray, R.M., O'keane, V., 2004. Effects of long-term prolactin-raising antipsychotic medication on bone mineral density in patients with schizophrenia. The British Journal of Psychiatry 184, 503-508.

Mockenhaupt, M., Messenheimer, J., Tennis, P., Schlingmann, J., 2005. Risk of Stevens–Johnson syndrome and toxic epidermal necrolysis in new users of antiepileptics. Neurology 64, 1134-1138.

Monaco, F., 2003. Classification of thyroid diseases: suggestions for a revision. The Journal of Clinical Endocrinology & Metabolism 88, 1428-1432.

Monaco, F., 2012. Thyroid Diseases. CRC Press.

Narayan, S.M., Stein, M.B., 2009. Do depression or antidepressants increase cardiovascular mortality? The absence of proof might be more important than the proof of absence. Journal of the American College of Cardiology 53, 959-961.

Nath, J., Sagar, R., 2001. Late-onset bipolar disorder due to hyperthyroidism. Acta Psychiatr. Scand. 104, 72-75.

O'Connell, M.B., Borgelt, L.M., Bowles, S.K., Vondracek, S.F., 2010. Drug-induced osteoporosis in the older adult. Aging health 6, 501-518.

Oakley, P.W., Whyte, I.M., Carter, G.L., 2001. Lithium toxicity: an iatrogenic problem in susceptible individuals. Australian and New Zealand journal of psychiatry 35, 833-840.

Osby, U., Brandt, L., Correia, N., Ekbom, A., Sparen, P., 2001. Excess mortality in bipolar and unipolar disorder in Sweden. Archives of general psychiatry 58, 844.

Package-Insert, CLOZARIL- clozapine tablet Novartis Pharmaceuticals Corporation, HUMAN PRESCRIPTION DRUG LABEL. National Library of Medicine (US).

Pantos, C., Mourouzis, I., Cokkinos, D.V., 2010. Thyroid hormone as a therapeutic option for treating ischaemic heart disease: from early reperfusion to late remodelling. Vascular pharmacology 52, 157-165.

Perros, P., Boelaert, K., Colley, S., Evans, C., Evans, R.M., Gerrard, B., Gilbert, J., Harrison, B., Johnson, S.J., Giles, T.E., 2014. Guidelines for the management of thyroid cancer. Clin. Endocrinol. (Oxf.) 81, 1-122.

Ponto, K.A., Zang, S., Kahaly, G.J., 2010. The tale of radioiodine and Graves' orbitopathy. Thyroid 20, 785-793.

Prange Jr, A., Haggerty Jr, J., Browne, J., Rice, J., 1990. Marginal hypothyroidism in mental illness: Preliminary assessments of prevalence and significance, Neuropsychopharmacology. Springer, pp. 352-361.

Ray, W.A., Meredith, S., Thapa, P.B., Meador, K.G., Hall, K., Murray, K.T., 2001. Antipsychotics and the risk of sudden cardiac death. Archives of General Psychiatry 58, 1161-1167.

Rezin, G.T., Amboni, G., Zugno, A.I., Quevedo, J., Streck, E.L., 2009. Mitochondrial dysfunction and psychiatric disorders. Neurochem. Res. 34, 1021-1029.

Ricken, R., Bermpohl, F., Schlattmann, P., Bschor, T., Adli, M., Monter, N., Bauer, M., 2012a. Long-term treatment with supraphysiological doses of thyroid hormone in affective disorders - effects on bone mineral density. J. Affect. Disord. 136, e89-94.

Ricken, R., Bermpohl, F., Schlattmann, P., Bschor, T., Adli, M., Mönter, N., Bauer, M., 2012b. Long-term treatment with supraphysiological doses of thyroid hormone in affective disorders—effects on bone mineral density. J. Affect. Disord. 136, e89-e94.

Rosenthal, L.J., Goldner, W.S., O'Reardon, J.P., 2011. T3 augmentation in major depressive disorder: safety considerations. American Journal of Psychiatry 168, 1035-1040.

Sachs, G.S., Printz, D.J., Kahn, D.A., Carpenter, D., Docherty, J.P., 2000. The expert consensus guideline series: medication treatment of bipolar disorder. Postgrad. Med. 1, 1-104.

Sawin, C.T., Geller, A., Wolf, P.A., Belanger, A.J., Baker, E., Bacharach, P., Wilson, P., Benjamin, E.J., D'Agostino, R.B., 1994. Low serum thyrotropin concentrations as a risk factor for atrial fibrillation in older persons. New England Journal of Medicine 331, 1249-1252.

Sbaihi, M., Kacem, A., Aroua, S., Baloche, S., Rousseau, K., Lopez, E., Meunier, F., Dufour, S., 2007. Thyroid hormone-induced demineralisation of the vertebral skeleton of the eel, Anguilla anguilla. General and comparative endocrinology 151, 98-107.

Schaffer, A., Isometsä, E.T., Tondo, L., H Moreno, D., Turecki, G., Reis, C., Cassidy, F., Sinyor, M., Azorin, J.M., Kessing, L.V., 2015. International Society for Bipolar Disorders Task Force on Suicide: meta-analyses and meta-regression of correlates of suicide attempts and suicide deaths in bipolar disorder. Bipolar disorders 17, 1-16.

Schelleman, H., Bilker, W.B., Kimmel, S.E., Daniel, G.W., Newcomb, C., Guevara, J.P., Cziraky, M.J., Strom, B.L., Hennessy, S., 2012.

Methylphenidate and risk of serious cardiovascular events in adults. American Journal of Psychiatry 169, 178-185.

Schett, G., David, J.-P., 2010. The multiple faces of autoimmune-mediated bone loss. Nature Reviews Endocrinology 6, 698-706.

Sinyor, M., Schaffer, A., Levitt, A., 2010. The sequenced treatment alternatives to relieve depression (STAR* D) trial: a review. The Canadian Journal of Psychiatry 55, 126-135.

Soto-Gomez, N., Anzueto, A., Waterer, G.W., Restrepo, M.I., Mortensen, E.M., 2013. Pneumonia: an arrhythmogenic disease? The American journal of medicine 126, 43-48.

Stagnaro-Green, A., Abalovich, M., Alexander, E., Azizi, F., Mestman, J., Negro, R., Nixon, A., Pearce, E.N., Soldin, O.P., Sullivan, S., 2011. Guidelines of the American Thyroid Association for the diagnosis and management of thyroid disease during pregnancy and postpartum. Thyroid 21, 1081-1125.

Stamm, T.J., Lewitzka, U., Sauer, C., Pilhatsch, M., Smolka, M.N., Koeberle, U., Adli, M., Ricken, R., Scherk, H., Frye, M.A., 2014. Supraphysiologic doses of levothyroxine as adjunctive therapy in bipolar depression: a randomized, double-blind, placebo-controlled study. The Journal of clinical psychiatry 75, 162-168.

Stork, C., Renshaw, P., 2005. Mitochondrial dysfunction in bipolar disorder: evidence from magnetic resonance spectroscopy research. Molecular psychiatry 10, 900-919.

Sugitani, I., Fujimoto, Y., 2011. Effect of postoperative thyrotropin suppressive therapy on bone mineral density in patients with papillary thyroid carcinoma: a prospective controlled study. Surgery 150, 1250-1257.

Sun, X., Jun-Feng, W., Tseng, M., Young, L.T., 2006. Downregulation in components of the mitochondrial electron transport chain in the postmortem frontal cortex of subjects with bipolar disorder. Journal of psychiatry & neuroscience: JPN 31, 189.

Talaeipour, A., Shirazi, M., Kheirandish, Y., Delrobaie, A., Jafari, F., Dehpour, A., 2014. Densitometric evaluation of skull and jaw bones after administration of thyroid hormones in rats. Dentomaxillofacial Radiology.

Tanner, M., Culling, W., 2003. Clozapine associated dilated cardiomyopathy. Postgraduate medical journal 79, 412-413.

Thanacoody, H.R., Thomas, S.H., 2003. Antidepressant poisoning. Clinical medicine 3, 114-118.

Toft, A.D., 2001. Subclinical hyperthyroidism. N. Engl. J. Med. 345, 512-516.

Topliss, D.J., Eastman, C.J., 2004. 5: Diagnosis and management of hyperthyroidism and hypothyroidism. Med. J. Aust. 180, 186-194.
Tóth, G., Baska, F., Schretner, A., Rácz, Á., Noszál, B., 2013. Site-specific basicities regulate molecular recognition in receptor binding: in silico docking of thyroid hormones. European Biophysics Journal 42, 721-730.
Trzepacz, P.T., Klein, I., Roberts, M., Greenhouse, J., Levey, G.S., 1989. Graves' disease: an analysis of thyroid hormone levels and hyperthyroid signs and symptoms. The American journal of medicine 87, 558-561.
van der Heyden, J.T., Docter, R., van Toor, H., Wilson, J.H., Hennemann, G., Krenning, E.P., 1986. Effects of caloric deprivation on thyroid hormone tissue uptake and generation of low-T3 syndrome. American Journal of Physiology - Endocrinology and Metabolism 251, E156-E163.
Vestergaard, P., 2008. Skeletal effects of central nervous system active drugs: anxiolytics, sedatives, antidepressants, lithium and neuroleptics. Current Drug Safety 3, 185-189.
Vieweg, W.V.R., Wood, M.A., 2004. Tricyclic antidepressants, QT interval prolongation, and torsade de pointes. Psychosomatics 45, 371-377.
Villani, S., Weitzel, W.D., 1979. Secondary mania. Arch. Gen. Psychiatry 36, 1031.
Wall, J.R., Lahooti, H., 2010. Pathogenesis of thyroid eye disease—does autoimmunity against the TSH receptor explain all cases. Endokrynol. Pol. 61, 222-227.
Wassen, F., Moerings, E., van Toor, H., Hennemann, G., Everts, M., 2000. Thyroid hormone uptake in cultured rat anterior pituitary cells: effects of energy status and bilirubin. Journal of endocrinology 165, 599-606.
Watts, N., Bilezikian, J., Camacho, P., Greenspan, S., Harris, S., Hodgson, S., Kleerekoper, M., Luckey, M., McClung, M., Pollack, R., 2010. American Association of Clinical Endocrinologists Medical Guidelines for Clinical Practice for the diagnosis and treatment of postmenopausal osteoporosis. Endocr. Pract. 16, 1-37.
Woolcott, J.C., Richardson, K.J., Wiens, M.O., Patel, B., Marin, J., Khan, K.M., Marra, C.A., 2009. Meta-analysis of the Impact of 9 Medication Classes on Falls in Elderly PersonsMedications and Falls in Elderly Persons. Archives of Internal Medicine 169, 1952-1960.
Yatham, L.N., Kennedy, S.H., Parikh, S.V., Schaffer, A., Beaulieu, S., Alda, M., O'Donovan, C., MacQueen, G., McIntyre, R.S., Sharma, V., 2013. Canadian Network for Mood and Anxiety Treatments (CANMAT) and International Society for Bipolar Disorders (ISBD) collaborative update of CANMAT guidelines for the management of patients with bipolar disorder: update 2013. Bipolar disorders 15, 1-44.

Yazdani, K., Lippmann, M., Gala, I., 2002. Fatal pancreatitis associated with valproic acid: Review of the literature. Medicine 81, 305-310.

Yip, K., Yeung, W., 2007. Lithium overdose causing non-convulsive status epilepticus-the importance of lithium levels and the electroencephalography in diagnosis. HONG KONG MEDICAL JOURNAL 13, 471.

Zamani, A., Omrani, G.R., Nasab, M.M., 2009. Lithium's effect on bone mineral density. Bone 44, 331-334.

Made in the USA
Middletown, DE
30 September 2018